Praise for *THE HEALING POWER OF ESSENTIAL OILS*

"In *The Healing Power of Essential Oils*, Dr. Z provides a cutting-edge and evidence-based approach to using essential oils. He astutely portrays how to prepare a variety of remedies. His well-written and detailed information makes this book a must-read for every essential oil user. Well done!"

—*STEVEN MASLEY, MD, FAHA, FACN, FAAFP, CNS,*
author of The Better Brain Solution

"If you're confused by conflicting claims about essential oils, pick up this book now and get the unbiased, evidence-based information you're seeking. *The Healing Power of Essential Oils* will become your favorite go-to guide if you're serious about using these health-boosting oils safely, smartly, and effectively."

—*KELLYANN PETRUCCI, MS, ND,* New York Times *bestselling author of* Dr. Kellyann's Bone Broth Diet *and* The 10-Day Belly Slimdown

"Amazing, captivating, and practical! This book is a must-have addition to your family health library. Not only does Dr. Z give us the history of essential oils, he gives us the recipes to help with ailments from A to Z. If you want to know how essential oils can help your family with pain, infection, fatigue, digestion, and many other chronic ailments, look no further than this essential oil bible!"

—*DR. PETER OSBORNE, author of the international bestseller* No Grain, No Pain

"Simply put, this is the best, most honest, clear, trustable, scientifically sound, and spiritually uplifting book on essential oils that you'll find. Dr. Eric Zielinski has done the near impossible. Armed with a researcher's mind, a caring heart, and an unstoppable faith, he has taken this beautifully important yet complex topic and made it accessible for everyone. Indeed, if you have been at all intrigued by essential oils, you have probably noticed that there is so much confusion and so many conflicting viewpoints put forth by experts. The good news is Dr. Z is a refreshing and compelling new thought leader in the time-honored field of aromatherapy. *The Healing Power of Essential Oils* clears things up and brings it all together—body, mind, heart, and soul. The science geek in you will be very satisfied, while the home-based healer in you will love the easy-to-understand and practical recommendations. You will know so much more about these special medicines than you ever knew you needed to know! So whether you're a professional or one of the countless numbers of people who've been captivated by the magic of essential oils, please consider this your cornerstone book, reference manual, and inspirational how-to guide all in one. I couldn't recommend *The Healing Power of Essential Oils* more highly."

—MARC DAVID, *founder of the Institute for the Psychology of Eating and author of* Nourishing Wisdom *and* The Slow Down Diet

"We've come full circle in medicine and are beginning to understand the incredible potency of plants. The essential oils of a plant are the true treasure of nature and Dr. Zielinski has brought this wisdom forth in a salient and accessible way. This book should be in every house and be used frequently."

—PEDRAM SHOJAI, OMD, *founder of Well.org and* New York Times *bestselling author of* The Urban Monk *and* The Art of Stopping Time

"Essential oils are everywhere these days; unfortunately, solid, evidence-based information on how to properly use them isn't as easy to find. Dr. Z is not afraid to dive into the research and tackle the hard and often confusing topics, which is exactly the reason I have come to look to him as one of my most trusted sources of natural health information. This book is sure to become one of the most dog-eared members of my essential oil library!"

—JILL WINGER, *ThePrairieHomestead.com*

The
HEALING POWER
of ESSENTIAL OILS

Soothe Inflammation, Boost Mood,
Prevent Autoimmunity, and Feel Great in Every Way

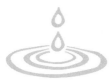

Eric Zielinski, D.C.

HARMONY
BOOKS · NEW YORK

Published in the United States by Harmony Books, an imprint of the Crown Publishing Group, a division of Penguin Random House LLC, New York.
crownpublishing.com

Harmony Books is a registered trademark, and the Circle colophon is a trademark of Penguin Random House LLC.

Library of Congress Cataloging-in-Publication Data

Names: Zielinski, Eric, author.
Title: The healing power of essential oils / Eric Zielinski, D.C.
Description: First edition. | New York : Harmony Books, [2018]
Identifiers: LCCN 2017046123| ISBN 9781524761363 (paperback) | ISBN 9781524761370 (ebook)
Subjects: LCSH: Aromatherapy—Popular works. | Essences and essential
   oils—Therapeutic use—Popular works. | BISAC: HEALTH & FITNESS /
   Alternative Therapies. | HEALTH & FITNESS / Healing. | HEALTH & FITNESS /
   Aromatherapy.
Classification: LCC RM666.A68 Z54 2018 | DDC 615.3/219—dc23
LC record available at https://lccn.loc.gov/2017046123

ISBN 978-1-5247-6136-3
Ebook ISBN 978-1-5247-6137-0

Printed in the United States of America

Book design by Lauren Dong
Cover design by Alane Gianetti
Cover photographs: (top to bottom) bigacis/Shutterstock; Daniel Hurst Photography/Moment/Getty Images; Inga Spence/Photolibrary/Getty Images; Botamochy/Shutterstock

10 9 8 7 6 5

First Edition

Sabrina Ann, if it weren't for you this book would not exist. You are one of the most talented people that I have ever met, and your contribution to this book was priceless. You are also one of the most giving people that I know, and I can think of no one else I'd rather do life with.

Esther, Isaiah, Elijah, and Isabella—thank you for your love, support, and patience during all of those long days and nights when Daddy was away working on this manuscript. My hope and prayer is that you come to realize it was all worth it because of the people we were able to help (together)!

I am eternally grateful to God for giving you all to me.

CONTENTS

PREFACE

Then I heard the voice of the Lord, saying, "Whom shall I send, and who will go for Us?" Then I said, "Here am I. Send me!" He said, "Go, and tell this people . . ."

—ISAIAH 6:8–9

've always been that guy to step up and do what needed to be done. I can remember being a kid and helping my elderly neighbors by shoveling their snow, not because my parents forced me, but because I wanted to. It made me feel good. And it still does. If I see a need, I try my best to fill it, especially when it involves people.

When I became a Christian, this part of me got amplified. Early on, I stumbled upon Isaiah 6:8–9 and I remember raising my hands in prayer, mimicking the prophet's words: "Here I am, Lord, send me!" I cried out, "I don't care what it is, I just want to do my part!" That prayer has proven to be the impetus for my biblical health ministry, my career, and notably my focus on educating people how to use essential oils therapeutically.

I'm actually a late bloomer when it comes to using essential oils. In fact, my wife, Sabrina, who has been using them since the early 1990s, tried to alert me to their power several times before I finally had my epiphany. I'll confess, as recently as a few years back I marginalized essential oils as the "smelly stuff" that Mama Z used every morning.

Thankfully, back in 2013 a client commissioned me to write a series of public health reports about essential oils. Supporting myself as a medical writer at the time, I was forced to take a second look.

That's when I had my "aha" moment. I got lost in the literature. On studying countless peer-reviewed studies, I was floored when I read the clinical research that supported the efficacy of essential oils as a viable option to treat chronic conditions like cancer, hypertension, obesity, and type 2 diabetes, not to mention mental illnesses like addiction, anxiety, depression, and stress. Whoa!

Suddenly, all of those too-good-to-be-true stories I had read online started to sound more plausible.

Excited about my newfound research, I told Mama Z about the potential role that essential oils can play in healing the body and preventing disease. She looked at me with those all-too-familiar "I told you so" eyes, and I knew that I had some catching up to do. So the journey began.

FOUR INVALUABLE LESSONS

As I pored over the research, it became glaringly clear that the articles I read in the blogosphere discussing essential oils and the information in the medical journals didn't jibe. Additionally, the blogs conflicted heavily with one another. Truthfully, it's a confusing mess out there, which explains the sheer number of people who regularly come to me unsure about how to use essential oils in the right way. Millions of people visit my website and social media pages every year to learn about essential oils. There are four reasons why I suspect this is so.

First, a vast majority of bloggers are simply not trained as public health researchers, medical writers, or aromatherapists and have no business teaching about the therapeutic nature of essential oils. Telling your personal healing story is one thing. Presenting yourself as a trained expert is quite another.

Second, most of the information in the blogosphere is woefully biased. As a public health researcher, I've been trained to sniff out bias a mile away—especially when there's a potential financial incentive at play. It's challenging to find statistically sound articles about essential oils without seeing banner ads for the very product that is being written about all over the website.

Third, there are huge chasms separating different factions of the essential oils industry, and things have a tendency to get ugly. These are the main players in the field:

- Aromatherapists
- Bloggers
- Chemists
- Governing agencies like the Food and Drug Administration (FDA)
- Health care providers (MDs, DOs, etc.)
- Network marketers
- Researchers
- Suppliers and manufacturers

Examples of these conflicts abound: Aromatherapists and multilevel marketing distributors are continually at odds with each other, disagreeing about the most fundamental principles of how to use essential oils therapeutically; chemists are often in disagreement with clinical researchers because they view essential oils through differing lenses; and consumers are always concerned as to whether manufacturers are supplying high-quality, pure oils. Moreover, governing agencies increasingly restrict the use of specific language across the field because essential oils are not approved "drugs," and therefore organizations and individuals that sell them for profit cannot make claims that they can heal the body, cure disease, or even have an effect on the structure/function of the body.

Finally, I observed that many doctors and pharmacists are leery of advising their patients about how to use essential oils, which makes patients nervous about potential contraindications and drug interactions. It would be untrue to say that medical doctors and pharmacists are not in favor of using alternative therapies, but because aromatherapy is not a topic that they learn about in school, they have no basis for discussing it with their patients unless they have studied the topic on their own. As I mentioned earlier, essential oils have yet to be approved by the FDA to prevent or treat disease, thus placing medical professionals in a sticky situation. They can neither confirm nor deny the therapeutic use of essential oils because it is out of their scope of practice.

DISCOVERING MY CALLING

The more I learned about the friction within the essential oils industry, the more I yearned to bring together thought leaders representing each group to lay aside their differences. With my friend Jill Winger from ThePrairieHomestead.com at the helm as my cohost, the idea behind the Essential Oils Revolution® online summit was born in June of 2014.

We decided to host a free online conference, commonly referred to as a "tele-summit," so we could provide interviews with these experts to a mass audience. Similar to live streaming YouTube videos, we created a website that acted like a conference meeting space. People from all over the globe could join for free and, from the comfort of their home, watch a series of interviews from experts representing nearly every sector of the essential oils community. Online health summits have been around for a while, but none about oils had really taken off because they tended to be a sales pitch to sell essential oils. To remedy this, we eliminated what public health researchers call financial or "brand bias" and ensured that every interview we conducted was nonbranded, meaning that even the slightest mention of the interviewee's favorite essential oil brand(s) was not permitted.

We set out to do what people told me was impossible because of the overwhelming animosity within the essential oils industry. With the exception of my loving, supportive wife, nearly everyone I spoke to said that we wouldn't be able to convene aromatherapists, bloggers, chemists, researchers, and health care professionals under "one roof" to talk about essential oils.

After nearly a year of rejected offers, criticism, and negativity from countless leaders within each camp, Jill and I proudly launched the Essential Oils Revolution on May 11, 2015. We carefully selected panelists to offer insight on different subjects related to their particular expertise and covered a gamut of topics from safety guidelines to cooking with oils to a myriad of health conditions, including cancer, autoimmune conditions, chronic fatigue, and weight loss.

More than 165,000 people from more than twenty countries participated in that first summit, which proved to be one of the largest online events of its kind. We received thousands of comments and emails from our online followers, and it became clear that most essential oil consumers were looking for an evidence-based, nonbranded resource to teach them about essential oils for their health concerns. People were not only desperate for help, they were uncertain where to go because of all the bias and conflicting information out there on the Internet.

The love and appreciation that came through those emails literally changed my life, and the experience of hosting the summit and helping folks improve their lives with essential oils actually shifted the entire focus of my career.

Truth be told, I had never intended to leave my career as a public health clinical researcher and medical writer. I never set out to be the online "essential oil guy." After seeing the obvious need, however, it seemed pretty clear that God was calling my wife and me to be that reliable resource that people were so desperately seeking to prevent and treat disease.

The book you are reading is the result of this calling. What you're holding in your hands is the best-of-the-best from my telesummits and literally thousands of hours of personal research and study. This book was crafted to be your go-to resource for all things related to using essential oils safely and effectively, and to empower you to approach the primary common health concerns affecting most people today.

I invite you to join me as I continue my journey to master the art and science of essential oils. I hope you enjoy the personal anecdotes as well as validating scientific research, and find my DIY hacks and recipes useful in your own quest to experience radiant health!

Introduction

The thief comes only to steal and kill and destroy. I came that they may have life and have it abundantly.

—JOHN 10:10

We know more about nutrition and health now than we ever have before. Yet nearly every single American is taking a supplement and/or a pharmaceutical medicine. Why, if we are so advanced in our health knowledge, are we also unhealthier than ever?

Put simply, it's because we've left nature out of the equation. God has provided us with what we need to be truly healthy. Need more vitamin D? Go out in the sun! Lacking vitamin C? Eat some limes! Need to improve your digestive health? Eat fermented foods! Have a cold, headache, or back pain? Use plant-based medicine such as essential oils!

There is a verse in Revelation (22:2) that reads: "Then the angel showed me a river of the water of life, as clear as crystal, flowing from the throne of God and of the Lamb, down the middle of the great street of the city. On each side of the river stood the tree of life, bearing twelve crops of fruit, yielding its fruit every month. And the leaves of the tree are for the healing of the nations."

I can think of no other substance on earth that epitomizes this Bible scripture more than essential oils, and I have come to see essential oils as a fundamental tool for achieving biblical health. They are the very essence of trees and plants, and they are vehicles of healing. And, in my opinion, they are also a cornerstone of a truly healthy life.

A CLOSER LOOK AT HEALTH

Health is a state of complete physical, mental and social well-being and not merely the absence of disease or infirmity.[1]

—WORLD HEALTH ORGANIZATION

Do you consider yourself a healthy person?

I'm not talking about the mere "absence of disease," as the World Health Organization (WHO) puts it in its definition of health. I'm asking if you are *really* well—physically, mentally, and socially. Biblical health is not a list of "thou shalt nots." It's an overarching concept that it is your God-given right to have and enjoy the abundant life that Christ refers to in John 10:10. Having an abundant life means that you enjoy the fullest expression of health in all areas of your life: spiritual, physical, mental, emotional, financial, occupational, and social. Every area of your life is connected to all the others. Like a chain, you are only as strong as your weakest link. If your physical body isn't performing how it should, it's going to weigh you down emotionally and cause strain in your relationships. If your job isn't going well or you aren't working to your full potential, it's going to impact your financial health and your mental health by raising your stress levels.

Again, let me ask you: Do you consider yourself a healthy person?

Consider writing your answer in the margin here or in your journal if you're taking notes as you read this book. Periodically, go back to this question and answer honestly. I'd be curious to see how your response changes as your understanding of health and healing evolves because of what you learn in this book. At its core, this health journey is about balance. The foods you eat, the drinks you consume, the supplements you take, the medicines you use, the thoughts you think, the emotions you carry around, the feelings you have about your job, your financial practices, the stressors you allow in your life—all of these contribute to or diminish your experience of an abundant life.

You want to find a point of equilibrium in each of the seven areas so that you don't feel off-kilter. Interestingly, I have discovered that using essential oils can help you find this balance, and I will show you how throughout this book.

MY PATH TO WELLNESS

As a kid, I never dreamed that I would one day be helping people restore their health. I didn't think much about health at all, honestly, apart from considering myself pretty healthy because I didn't suffer from any serious, life-threatening conditions like cancer. As I look back on my life, however, I see a different picture because I certainly didn't enjoy the "complete physical, mental and social well-being" that the WHO refers to.

My health issues surfaced soon after birth. At just a few months old, I was so "chunky," as my mom lovingly puts it, that my pediatrician advised that she feed me 2% milk because the formula I was exclusively drinking was making me fat. I haven't checked the *Guinness Book of World Records* to confirm, but I'm confident that I would have earned the dubious distinction of being one of the youngest people ever to be placed on a "diet"!

This was the beginning of a childhood marred by misguided advice from medical professionals for seemingly normal health concerns.

My mom tells me that I started to get sick when I went to preschool. Like many children today, I had frequent bouts of tonsillitis and numerous rounds of antibiotics, which led to a tonsillectomy and adenoidectomy when I was in elementary school. About that time I also started to develop anxiety and to battle stress and a variety of fears. To address a chronic stammering condition that worsened as my social phobias progressed, I began a seven-year relationship with a speech therapist in first grade.

By the time I reached middle school, I started to withdraw inwardly. My social awkwardness skyrocketed as cystic acne scarred my face. My dermatologist suggested a solution: take Accutane, a drug that was originally developed for chemotherapy but later commonly prescribed for skin conditions—and that has been linked to birth defects, depression, and suicidal ideation.

In high school, chronic pains in my joints started to develop and recurring gastrointestinal issues like gas and indigestion made my life quite uncomfortable nearly every day. Insecurity and fear prevented me from chasing a childhood dream of moving out of state and going away to college. Taking the easy way out, I chose to attend a local university and studied English literature because it came easy to me.

At one point during my college career, it dawned on me that I wasn't living my own life. I was letting other people's expectations of me and the status quo determine how I lived. This caused a deep sense of purposelessness that I'll never forget. It was like I was falling into a black hole, and every single day that went by, the light around me got dimmer and dimmer. Not long thereafter depression settled in and I fell into the habit of taking over-the-counter medications, alcohol, and street narcotics to numb the pain.

As I stayed out until all hours of the night partying and masking my inner torment with reckless living, my energy levels plummeted, and I got to the point where I needed a pot of coffee and a pack of cigarettes to get through the day. And I wasn't even out of college yet!

By the time I was twenty-two, I had reached rock bottom and started to ponder taking my own life. It was then that I put my faith in a higher power, and my life was forever transformed. The day that I asked God to free me from all of my addictions seems like yesterday. After I had failed numerous times to quit smoking and drugs, God delivered me overnight. No withdrawals. No detoxing. Nothing. It was like my body was given a second chance. Like I was literally born again. Depression and suicidal ideation disappeared, and I had a renewed vigor for life and a hope that I truly had a purpose to fulfill on this planet.

To be clear, not every symptom immediately evaporated, as if God had said, "Poof! You're healed!" The litany of health issues that I described—the gut issues, the aches and pains, and the acne—still lingered. At first, I was confused. "Come on, God," I negotiated. "You healed me of the other stuff; why not these?"

You see, if I had been healed of everything all at once, I don't think that I'd have the appreciation for health and wellness that I do today. Hitting my rock bottom and then fighting my way back to health one issue at a time helped me develop patience, character, and perseverance—qualities I value in myself and try to instill in my children every day.

EXPERIENCING YOUR OWN TRANSFORMATION

I learned that my health was my own responsibility—not that of my doctor, my spouse, or anyone else. I was empowered by the revelation that health is an act of self-love and not something that I should focus on merely to be free of sickness. I also realized that I couldn't take *anyone's* word at face value. Paul's admonishment to the Thessalonian church to "test all things and to hold fast to that which is good" became my guiding principle. Lastly, I came to see that we're all under construction and that I needed to give myself grace whenever I missed the mark.

In his book *From Within I Rise,* T. F. Hodge puts it this way: "You cannot build a dream on a foundation of sand. To weather the test of storms, it must be cemented in the heart with uncompromising conviction."[2] I urge you to find your own conviction to become truly healthy, whatever that inspiration may be, and act on it.

Even if you don't feel that conviction at this very moment, get started today on improving your health. As you learn how to do that in these pages, focus on the low-hanging fruit—do those things that are easiest for you to implement right away to get some quick wins, which will increase your conviction. Take it line by line. Here a little, there a little. If you use the fundamental principles of this book to adopt an essential oils–based, holistic health lifestyle, you will never look back.

GETTING THE MOST OUT OF THIS BOOK

Are you overwhelmed by all of the information out there about essential oils? You're not alone! Many of the sources that you may be reading use fear tactics or overstate potential therapeutic efficacy to convince you to follow their advice (or buy their products). This misguided and often conflicting information leaves a trail of bewildered consumers who are confused about how to use essential oils safely and effectively.

It's with this in mind that I offer you four strategies to get the most out of this book:

1. Don't overanalyze.
2. Quiet the noise.
3. Focus on the low-hanging fruit.
4. Remember biochemical individuality.

1. Don't Overanalyze

Two phrases I learned during my short stint in the sales world were "paralysis by analysis" and "ignorance on fire."

We were taught not to overthink things, which is a surefire way to feel that you're not prepared to approach a customer and to make you freeze up before you ever get the chance to land the sale—in other words, paralysis by analysis. The most successful salespeople, on the other hand, tend to act before they think through all of the potential objections and have a much higher close rate—demonstrating ignorance on fire.

I have observed that many online health consumers fall into the paralysis by analysis trap. They have a tendency to agonize about the details and quickly become overwhelmed—and then are too afraid to move forward. To be fair, I can understand why. Health is a serious issue and people's lives are at stake. Not to mention that the information out there in the blogosphere is anything but consistent.

What's the solution? Don't overanalyze! I don't mean that you should try essential oils willy-nilly. Commit to educating yourself, but learn at your own pace and implement the recommendations offered in this book only as you're comfortable. This isn't a race.

2. Quiet the Noise

When you first start using essential oils it can be tempting to read everything you can get your hands on—from your new essential oils distributor to your favorite blogger, your medical doctor, and even your Facebook friend who fancies herself an essential oils expert. Maintaining a scientific focus is important, but feeling that you must read everything you can and interrogate everyone you know, until you're completely overwhelmed, can be counterproductive.

A practical way to move forward is to limit your teachers to just two or three when you're first starting out. This is not to say that you shouldn't get a second opinion, but resist the urge to get a fourth, fifth, or sixth opinion, or else you're likely to hear such conflicting information that you won't know what to do.

Do your research and vet your sources by making sure they have valid credentials. When I first started learning about essential oils, I didn't follow food bloggers. I sought out aromatherapists, chemists, and health care professionals with ample experience using essential oils in their research and practices.

When you find a quality resource, let your guard down and receive what's being shared with you, just as a student does with her teacher. Then, when you have the basics down pat, you'll be better prepared to venture into the Wild West and comb through the vast array of Internet resources!

3. Focus on Low-Hanging Fruit

Implementing essential oils into your daily routine is more than a fad; it's a way of life. Even though the journey to health is a marathon, not a sprint, quick wins are a must because they create confidence, which is the foundation for long-term success.

This is why focusing on the lowest-hanging fruit makes the most sense. Set aside the advanced aromatherapy concepts and formulas until a later date when your knowledge and confidence are built up. Do something quick and easy first, like the Essential Oils Daily Practice in chapter 5 (page 86). It's all there, easily spelled out, ripe for the picking.

Making your own hand sanitizer is another great place to start. Everyone seems to be using the commercially produced stuff, and yet it couldn't be more toxic. Want a quick win? Toss the hand sanitizer and make your own. You can get everything you need on Amazon, it costs only a few bucks, and it will take you just a few minutes to make a dozen batches. Check out my recipe on page 144.

4. Remember Biochemical Individuality

By far the hardest concept for new essential oil users to grasp is biochemical individuality. In a nutshell: What works for me, a thirty-seven-year-old Caucasian male with Polish and Sicilian ancestry, will not necessarily work for a seventy-five-year-old African-American female. Our physiologies are as unique as our fingerprints. There simply is no one-size-fits-all approach to health care. There are always multiple ways to achieve the effects you seek, just as there's more than one way to paint a wall.

This trips people up because we've been indoctrinated by the medical community to believe that a standardized approach to health care is ideal: Are you sick? Take this pill that everyone else is taking. You all have the same sickness, so why shouldn't you all take the same remedy?

This seems logical, but don't forget that it presupposes that all the variables are the same. You may all have the same sickness. But is everything else the same? What about your weight, race, gender, comorbidities, and contributing factors like stress, diet, and drugs you are currently taking?

We all have different biochemical makeups, and you need to find what works for you.

Lavender is the perfect example. Traditionally a sedative, this popular oil can have the opposite effect on certain people and act more like a stimulant. This is why I'll always suggest that you try multiple oils before giving up and running to the pharmacy—you never know what will work for you. You need to give your search time, and it takes practice.

Resist any claim that says, "There's an oil for that." This isn't true, because we're all different!

A GIFT TO HELP YOU ON YOUR JOURNEY

The therapeutic use of essential oils doesn't have to be complicated. Yes, you could dive into some advanced concepts, like chemistry, blending, and interpreting scientific studies, but you don't have to worry about any of that with this book. I have painstakingly taken out all of the guesswork and have tried my best to distill everything down to manageable bite-sized pieces.

Remember, learning a new skill takes time and practice, and digesting the material presented in this book is no exception. Let me suggest that you make a hot cup of herbal tea, cozy up in your favorite chair, and begin the wonderful journey. Trust me, it'll be worth it!

To help you along the journey, I have created a series of demo videos showing you how to prepare several of my essential oil blends. Each of the videos also contains extra insight into the strategies and information covered in this book. You can access those videos for free at HealingPowerOfEssentialOils.com.

Part 1
Essential Oils Revolution

I alone cannot change the world, but I can cast a stone across the waters to create many ripples.

—MOTHER TERESA

Using natural therapies such as essential oils is about so much more than physical healing. It's about empowering yourself to transform yourself and your life.

Throughout my life, being sick was a constant for me and, like many people today, I was a victim of misguided medical advice. I was woefully unprepared to manage my own health. In fact, I felt that my only problem was that I needed more antibiotics and other prescription drugs—I literally expected (and often requested) drugs every time I visited my primary care physician. Evidently, I'm not alone.

A Medscape report shares a shocking story of one physician who blames patients for the misuse of medical treatments because of the sheer volume of people "who flood urgent care centers seeking care for run-of-the-mill ailments such as 'simple ankle sprains, sore throats or diarrhea for one day, sunburns—the list goes on. None of us would even consider seeing a doctor for such common and trivial matters,' the physician stated in an interview. 'I see about 50 patients a day, and easily 75 percent of them have no business seeing a physician. And 80 percent of those patients are expecting antibiotics.'"[1]

Can you relate?

At its core, my work to spread research-backed information on essential oils is designed to educate families that they don't need to visit their health care provider for every little ailment. At the very least, you'll be armed with enough information to question your health care provider about alternatives before taking a prescription drug or having a procedure done. Hopefully, you'll have a natural solution or two in your tool belt so that you can handle some things all by yourself! Even better, thanks to the preventative effect of essential oils, perhaps you'll have fewer ailments that need remedies in the first place.

This is one of the many reasons I'm so passionate about essential oils—they empower us to manage our own health. With essential oils, you can finally get a better night's sleep, reduce stress, boost your mood, clear brain fog, balance your hormones, and ease pain—and that's just the beginning! Are you ready to get started?

1

Fundamentals of Aromatherapy

Your oils have a pleasing fragrance, Your name is like purified oil; Therefore the maidens love you. . . . How beautiful is your love, my sister, my bride! How much better is your love than wine, And the fragrance of your oils Than all kinds of spices!

—SONG OF SOLOMON 1:3, 4:10

Imagine yourself walking through a beautiful garden. After brushing up against a rose, you faintly smell the floral scent. You bend over to get a better whiff and encounter an aroma that stops you in your tracks. This, my friend, is the essential oil.

Or, imagine making homemade lemonade as a refreshing treat after working in the garden on a hot summer day. When you've finished cutting all of the lemons and juicing them, you are pleasantly surprised to find your kitchen permeated with an uplifting, citrus aroma. This, too, is the essential oil.

Essential oils represent nature in its most concentrated form. They are extracted directly from the bark, flowers, fruit, leaves, nut, resin, or roots of a plant or tree, and just one drop contains a complex network of molecules that deliver myriad effects to the body. They are entirely, utterly natural.

Used medicinally for thousands of years through a variety of nonconcentrated forms, the true power of these oils is not in facilitating one-time therapeutic effects (as drugs do), but in addressing physiological disharmony and helping your body achieve the inner balance it needs to heal itself. And their power to facilitate healing is so effective that the scientific world has begun to take note—thousands of peer-reviewed articles published in databases around the world discuss their efficacy.

LAYING THE FOUNDATION

Before you dive into the therapeutic use of these precious plant-based compounds, you need to understand the basics. I welcome you along a journey that I hope will prove not only insightful but also empowering.

Think of growing your understanding of essential oils as a project similar to building a house. If the foundation isn't set properly, the entire structure will soon crumble, particularly when a storm hits. And storms always seem to hit at the most inopportune moments, don't they?

Using essential oils requires patience, study, and practice and should never be seen as a "quick fix" for your health problems. You need to learn how to use them properly. If you're not armed with the foundational principles of essential oils, you won't know what to do or where to turn for answers if the results aren't what you expect. You might give up on using natural solutions far too soon, or fall back into the prescription medication trap, even though many drugs have long-term consequences, including, for some, a risk of addiction.

When you take the information and instruction in this book to heart, I trust that this will never happen to you.

SETTING THE RECORD STRAIGHT

On coming to the house, they saw the child with his mother Mary, and they bowed down and worshiped him. Then they opened their treasures and presented him with gifts of gold, frankincense and myrrh.

—Matthew 2:11

While it's not an exhaustive study of the subject, consider this section my very best attempt to distill six thousand years of recorded use of essential oils down to a *Reader's Digest* version of aromatherapy history.

Are you ready?

OK, let's put first things first with a myth-buster that may shake up your essential oil theology: Jesus didn't use essential oils. It's actually one of the more pervasive delusions among lay people and students of biblical health. I can't tell you how many times I've heard people say, "If it's good enough for Baby Jesus, then it's good enough for me!"

Truth is, the magi gave the Christ child gold, frankincense, and myrrh *resins*. How do I know this? Because essential oils as we know them didn't exist back then—the essential oils that we use today require highly advanced distillation techniques that weren't yet invented.

Of course, crudely distilled alcoholic beverages have been around since our earliest recorded history—museums have three-thousand-year-old terra-cotta distillation apparatuses on display—but the likelihood that anyone could have extracted essential oils from plants is slim to none.

What we do know is that virtually every culture dating back to the beginning of time used aromatic plant materials in their sacred rituals as incense, in their body care as ointments and perfumes, and in their medicine as poultices, salves, and tinctures. Could Mary have created a healing salve or ointment from the frankincense resin that the magi gave her? Certainly. But she didn't use a drop of myrrh essential oil to cure Jesus of a sore throat. Big difference!

THE CLIFFSNOTES VERSION OF THE HISTORY OF AROMATHERAPY

Moreover, the Lord spoke to Moses, saying, "Take also for yourself the finest of spices: of flowing myrrh *five hundred shekels, and of fragrant* cinnamon *half as much, two hundred and fifty, and of fragrant* calamus *two hundred and fifty, and of* cassia *five hundred, according to the shekel of the sanctuary, and of* olive oil *a hint. You shall make of these a holy anointing oil, a perfume mixture, the work of a perfumer; it shall be a holy anointing oil.*

—Exodus 30:11–25

Burning leaves, resins, and other aromatic plant materials for incense has been a religious tradition throughout recorded history. As far as we can tell, these practices ushered in the dawn of aromatherapy.

The first records of essential oils as we know them today come from ancient Egypt, India, and, much later, Persia. Both Greece and Rome conducted extensive trade in aromatic oils and ointments with the Orient.[1] It's safe to assume that these products—not unlike the holy anointing oil recipe that God gave Moses—were extracts prepared by soaking flowers, leaves, resins, and roots in various fatty vegetable oils like olive and sesame.

It is presumed that fatty oils and alcohol were exclusively used to extract the essential oils from aromatic plants up until the golden age of Arab culture (eighth–thirteenth century AD), when a technique was developed using an alcohol solvent.[2] History tells us that Arabs were the first to distill ethyl alcohol from fermented sugar, which could have been used to replace vegetable oils to create aromatic extracts (more on the difference between extracts and essential oils to come).

The history books are in disagreement over the exact dates and to whom we should give credit for first inventing hydro (steam) distillation, but it seems fair to say that we can thank Arab alchemists from the ninth century AD. One of the first dated references to the "quintessence" of plants (i.e., essential oils) dates back to *The Book of Perfume Chemistry and Distillation* by Yakub al-Kindi (803–870).[3] Many credit Ibn-Sina, more commonly known as Avicenna (980–1037), for discovering distillation, but that's still debated. In either case, he has gone down in history as being the one of the first to document using essential oils in his practice, including an entire treatise on rose oil![4]

Fast-forward to early-twentieth-century France, when the renaissance of aromatherapy was birthed after chemist René-Maurice Gattefossé suffered a laboratory explosion and stumbled upon lavender essential oil as the remedy to heal the gas gangrene that ensued on his hand. Gattefossé devoted the remainder of his life to researching the therapeutic nature of essential oils and reported using many—such as chamomile, clove, lemon, and thyme, which were also used to disinfect surgical equipment and to treat infected wounds—on his patients during both world wars.[5] The science of aromatherapy was recorded in print with his seminal work *Aromatherapie: The Essential Oils—Vegetable Hormones.*

Commonly misunderstood today to refer solely to the inhalation of essential oils (i.e., diffusing, nebulizing, enjoying their aroma), the term *aromatherapy* is more properly defined as the therapeutic use of essential oils.

SCIENCEY INFORMATION FOR ESSENTIAL OIL GEEKS

Let's take a moment to walk through a couple of key terms, starting with the most fundamental of all: fixed oils and essential oils. You may wonder why the essential oils you've come in contact with don't seem all that, well, *oily*. That's because there are two different types of oils, which have different chemical (and, therefore, therapeutic) properties.

- **Fixed oils.** Also known as *expressed* or *fatty oils*, fixed oils are derived from both animals and plants. Common examples are cooking oils, including coconut, olive, and other vegetables oils that you see at the market. They contain fatty acids such as triglycerides, as well as certain phytochemicals, including vitamins, minerals, and a host of others. In contrast to volatile oils (aka *essential oils*), fixed oils do not evaporate (they will leave a stain on an absorbent surface), and thus cannot be distilled. Obtained by expression (the act of squeezing or using pressure) or extraction (drawing out using a solvent), fixed oils vary in consistency depending on the temperature and can be solid, semisolid, or liquid.[6]
- **Essential oils.** Also known as *volatile oils* because they evaporate readily, essential oils are the lipophilic ("fat loving"), hydrophobic ("water hating") *volatile organic compounds* that are found in aromatic plants. Meaning, they have the tendency to dissolve or combine with fats or lipids, while repelling or not mixing with water. Somewhat of a misnomer, essential oils aren't "oily" like the fixed, culinary oils just described, and they usually do not leave a residue when applied to your skin. They are generally insoluble in water but soluble in alcohol and fixed oils, and can dissolve fatty materials such as grease. Unlike fixed oils, they do not contain any nutritional content like vitamins or minerals.

Let's clear up another common misconception: Once referred to as "essential" because they were thought to represent the very essence of odor and flavor, essential oils are not "essential" for life at all.[7] However, though they may not be "necessary" for life, I can think of no other substance on the planet that I would consider essential to have in my medicine cabinet!

What gives these precious plant compounds their healing powers are the more than three hundred different aromatic molecules found in each bottle, and chemists are continually identifying more. These compounds contain physiological and pharmacological properties that affect nearly every organ and virtually every function necessary to human life.[8]

The amount of oil in each plant varies considerably—it takes more than three hundred pounds of rose petals, thirty pounds of lavender flowers, or forty-five lemons to fill just one of those itty-bitty 15 ml bottles of essential oil that you have in your home. Just think about how many tons of plant matter it must take to supply the world's growing need for these precious plant-based compounds!

The compounds contained in an essential oil are affected by how the oil is extracted and what part of the plant is used. While you don't necessarily need this information to buy and start using essential oils, reading it can help expand your understanding of these potent healers. And since this is a book that can live on your shelf for years, as you're ready to deepen your learning about essential oils, you can always revisit this section.

Thankfully, we are continually perfecting the manufacturing methods necessary to extract the volatile organic compounds from plants.

UNDERSTANDING ESSENTIAL OIL MANUFACTURING TO HELP YOU PURCHASE THE RIGHT PRODUCTS

Have you noticed that your favorite bottle of vanilla is not labeled as an oil, but an "absolute"? Yep! Same with jasmine and other plants that are too delicate to steam distill.

Or, have you seen the term CO2 on your bottle of turmeric or frankincense? These bottles look and even smell like essential oils, but they are different products because they were not steam distilled. And, because they were extracted differently than essential oils, they contain unique chemical properties, which lead to different therapeutic benefits and safety considerations.

The obstacle that all essential oil users have to overcome is that some companies mislabel their bottles and some sellers misrepresent their products. Even worse, I've encountered dozens of studies written by scientists who refer to the wrong products in their research.

Bottom line: Absolutes, CO2 extracts, and essential oils should not be used interchangeably. Most of the research we have is about essential oils, which is why I don't cover the medicinal uses of CO2 extracts in much detail in this book because they are still considered experimental.

So, to help you understand the differences among the various products on the market today, here is an overview of the primary extraction methods to be aware of before you start purchasing essential oils:

- **CO2 extraction.** Supercritical fluid extraction (SFE) uses supercritical carbon dioxide (sCO2), which is a fluid state where CO2 is held at or above its critical temperature and critical pressure. Not to get too deep into chemistry here; you're most likely familiar with CO2 being a gas at standard temperature and pressure (STP), or dry ice when frozen. In its supercritical, fluid state, it has an uncanny ability to perform as a commercial and industrial solvent. Unlike other commonly used toxic solvents, like hexane, CO2 is safe and environmentally friendly. The resulting extract is currently all the rage in the aromatherapy community.
- **Distillation.** Primarily produced with steam, essential oils can also be water and steam distilled as well as steam vacuum distilled. Let me help you visualize the process: Steam from boiling water comes into contact with biomass (lavender flowers, sandalwood, cinnamon bark, etc.), softens it, and breaks up the volatile organic compounds (VOCs). Now loose, the lipophilic/hydrophobic (nonpolar, or nonsoluble in water) VOCs then pass through a condenser wherein the steam separates them from the biomass that originally contained them. Also traveling with the steam are the lipidphobic/hydrophilic (polar,

or soluble in water) components of the plant. In the condenser, the steam is cooled and the polar constituents separate from the nonpolar constituents while sitting in a tube. The water is then separated from the oil, and what's left are hydrosols ("floral waters") and essential oils.

If you're keen on trying to do this yourself, you can pick up a home distiller kit for a few hundred bucks. It takes a little getting used to, but you'll find that you can make some high-quality oils from many of the herbs, shrubs, and trees you have in your backyard!

- **Enfleurage.** One of the most expensive ways to extract volatile organic compounds, enfleurage is used for fragile flowers such as jasmine. This is a labor-intensive process that is rarely used today; however, it is still interesting to note because of its historical significance. Enfleurage can take weeks to complete and essentially uses animal fat (pounded and coated onto glass) to extract the essential oils from delicate flowers. The end result is an oil/fat mixture known as a *pomade* that needs to be washed with alcohol to remove the fat. After the fat is removed, an extract containing volatile and nonvolatile principles is left, so it's referred to as an *absolute*.

- **Expression.** Primarily reserved for citrus peels, mechanical pressing (aka *cold pressing*) literally squeezes the volatile organic compounds out of the rind of a fruit. At one point in history, this was done by hand using a sponge to collect the oil, but those days are long gone. Citrus oils can also be steam distilled, but the aroma has a tendency to change considerably and the therapeutic properties are much different.

- **Solvent extraction.** A type of liquid-to-liquid extraction, this is what our biblical ancestors utilized to extract minuscule amounts of frankincense essential oil out of the resin by placing it in olive oil for a short time. Today, it is used for delicate flowers, such as rose, jasmine, and mimosa. The process has been expedited and much more of the volatile organic compounds can be extracted by using petroleum ether or chemical solvents like ethanol and hexane, all of which have safety concerns for us and for the environment. For this reason, safer alternatives like CO_2 extraction are becoming more popular. Solvent extraction produces a waxy, fatty substance known as a *concrete*. When the concrete is washed with alcohol, the fat is separated and the remaining end product, which contains volatile and nonvolatile compounds, is referred to as an *absolute*.

The various forms of extraction produce different types of products. I list below the most common plant products that fall within the scope of medicinal use of aromatic plants. Taking note of these differences and being an avid label reader will not only empower you to become a more informed consumer, it will also help ensure that you're spending your money on the right products to meet your health goals.

- **Absolutes.** A by-product of enfleurage and solvent extraction, absolutes are highly concentrated aromatic plant compounds that are widely used in the cosmetic and perfume industries as well as in the mental health field because of their uplifting aroma. The aroma generally resembles the actual plant that it was extracted from. Examples include rose, jasmine, and vanilla.
- **CO2 extracts.** CO2 extracts are still very experimental as few clinical trials have been conducted evaluating their safety and efficacy. That said, they are quite popular now in the aromatherapy community because, unlike with steam distillation, many more (medicinal) plant compounds are extracted during the process, no potentially harmful solvents are required, the oils are sometimes gentler to use on the skin, and their aromas are truer to the original plant than those of steam-distilled essential oils. Some of the more popular CO2 extracts are cannabis, turmeric, and vanilla.
- **Cold-pressed citrus oils.** Citrus oils that are expressed are much different from their steam-distilled counterparts. They are darker in color, they can stain clothing, and their aroma resembles the original peel much more closely. Technically speaking, citrus oils are not essential oils at all because they contain nonvolatile principals, but the aromatherapy and chemistry communities have made an exception to the rule. For more information on the safety differences (phototoxicity) between expressed and distilled citrus oils, see the

list of photosensitizing and nonphotosensitizing essential oils on pages 54 and 55.

- **Steam distilled essential oils.** Steam distillation often changes the aromatic compounds in the plant. The classic example is the distillation of German chamomile, when the chemical *matricin* is changed by the high-temperature steam to *chamazulene*. Not a bad thing necessarily, as both have anti-inflammatory properties, but it's important to note that the chemical contents (and therefore the specific therapeutic effects) of steam-distilled essentials oils are often different from those of the original plant. Look for labels that indicate whether the bottle contents have been steam distilled. Otherwise, you can never be sure how the product was extracted and whether or not it's truly an essential oil!
- **Extracts.** Similar to absolutes in that they contain volatile and nonvolatile principles, extracts are popular because they retain many of the same chemical properties of essential oils. Popular examples are cinnamon bark, clove, ginger, lemon, nutmeg, orange, peppermint, rose, spearmint, vanilla, and wintergreen. They are extracted using nonalcoholic solvents such as water, glycerin, and vinegar.
- **Hydrosols.** Also known as hydrolats, distillate waters, or floral waters, hydrosols contain the water-soluble compounds from distilled plants and contain a minuscule amount of essential oils. They are very safe to consume, and work wonderfully as spritzers and as fragrances for body care products. After you purchase hydrosols, be careful to refrigerate and use them speedily—they have a tendency to develop bacterial overgrowth and go rancid. Common examples on the market today include lavender, neroli, Roman chamomile, and rose.
- **Infused oils.** The by-product of submerging aromatic plant matter in a fixed oil for days or weeks, infused oil is reminiscent of what our ancestors would have used as perfume, anointing oils, or healing ointments.
- **Tinctures.** Using alcohol as the principal solvent to extract essential oils out of plants, tinctures are concentrated herbal remedies that have a long history of medicinal use. They are very easy to make, requiring only unflavored 80 to 90 proof vodka, some herbal biomass, a mason jar, and about two months to steep. Examples include arnica, St. John's wort, garlic, and echinacea.

PLANT PARTS THAT PRODUCE ESSENTIAL OILS

The other factor that contributes to the properties of an essential oil is the part of the plant that it was extracted from. I've fielded numerous questions from people about the origin of their essential oils. The following chart provides a quick overview of the plant parts that make up your favorite oils.

PLANT PARTS THAT PRODUCE ESSENTIAL OILS

PART	PLANT
Balsam, gum, and resin	Elemi, frankincense, galbanum, myrrh, Peru balsam
Bark	Cassia, cinnamon
Berries and fruit	Allspice, black pepper, juniper berry, *Litsea cubeba*
Flowers and leaves	Basil, catnip, clary sage, hyssop, lavender, lavandin, marjoram, Melissa (lemon balm), oregano, peppermint, rosemary, sage, spearmint, thyme
Flowers, petals, and buds	Chamomile, clove, helichrysum, jasmine, neroli, rose, ylang ylang
Leaves	Bay, cajuput, cinnamon, eucalyptus, geranium, myrtle, niaouli, patchouli, petitgrain, tea tree
Needles	Cypress, fir, Scotch pine, spruce
Peel/rind	Bergamot, lemon, lime, mandarin, sweet/wild orange, tangerine, yuzu
Roots	Angelica, ginger, spikenard, vetiver
Seeds	Anise, cardamom, carrot, coriander, cumin, dill, fennel, nutmeg, parsley
Wood	Cedarwood, palo santo, rosewood, sandalwood

From "The Parts of Plants That Produce Essential Oil," AromaWeb.com.

This information is not just for Trivial Pursuit buffs. It is important to consider the practical applications since essential oils derived from different parts of a plant can have very different uses and cautions. So, before you start using a particular oil to treat a specific condition, be sure you're using the right one for the purpose.

For example, cinnamon essential oil most commonly comes from the *Cinnamomum zeylanicum* tree. From there, either the inner bark or the leaves can be harvested for distillation. This should be indicated as either "cinnamon bark" or "cinnamon leaf" on the bottle. The bark and leaf oils each have their own chemical composition, which means they have very different medicinal properties.

Cinnamon leaf essential oil, for example, is steam distilled from cinnamon leaves, is yellowish in color, and contains high amounts of eugenol (68.6%–87.0%) and some cinnamaldehyde (0.6%–1.1%).

Cinnamon bark essential oil, on the other hand, is steam distilled from cinnamon bark, is reddish-brown in color, and contains mostly cinnamaldehyde (63.1%–75.7%) and much less eugenol (2.0%–13.3%).

Containing significantly more eugenol—a naturally occurring chemical with antibacterial and anti-inflammatory properties—cinnamon leaf is used widely to relieve pain and inflammation and to fight infectious agents. The bark is composed more of cinnamaldehyde and camphor, and its primary uses are as a potent antioxidant, antiviral, and antidiabetic.[9]

WHY DO ESSENTIAL OILS EXIST IN THE FIRST PLACE?

The function of volatile organic compounds in nature is not well understood. One obvious role is to give the plant its aroma—which attracts (or deters) pollinators, animals, and humans. Beyond this obvious benefit, the purposes that essential oils serve in nature have been debated for years.

Still, we can logically conjecture a few of the other reasons why plants might be endowed with precious essential oils:[10]

- To protect plants from herbivores and vectors like flies and mosquitoes—essential oils are generally quite bitter and many have an exceptional ability to repel insects.

- To protect plants from bacteria, fungi, and viruses—essential oils are supremely antimicrobial (a fact you'll hear me say over and over again in this book).
- To heal the plant from fungal infection, cuts, scrapes, and abrasions—essential oils are fantastic wound healers.

HOW ESSENTIAL OILS ARE USED IN THE INDUSTRIAL WORLD

Commercially, essential oils are used extensively as agrochemicals, fragrances, flavors, industrial cleaners, and pharmaceuticals. At first, you might be surprised to learn that the flavor industry is the top consumer of essential oils—even more than the aromatherapy community, which includes your favorite essential oil brand! But after you think about the sheer volume of colas and sodas, peppermint candies, and lemon bars that are consumed every day, this probably makes more sense. If there's a flavor or aroma in one of your favorite foods or household items, chances are you can thank an essential oil.

Here's a breakdown of the industries that use essential oils and the approximate percentage of all the essential oils on the market that you'll find in these products:[11]

- Food and flavors: 50%
- Fragrance: 25%
- Pharmaceutical: 20% (mostly used to flavor medicine, though menthol is used for nausea and stomach upset)
- Industrial: 3%
- Aromatherapy: only 2%

DECIPHERING THE SCIENTIFIC NAMES ON ESSENTIAL OIL BOTTLES

The botanical names on your bottles are important for a number of reasons, but mainly because they indicate similar chemical makeups among plants within the same species and sometimes genus, which can help narrow down how and when you should use certain essential oils. Essentially, it's all about chemistry.

Ready to jog your memory of the plant kingdom chart from grade school? Let's distill it to the most important takeaways that you need to become a savvy essential oil user.

- **Family:** The larger group (above genus) that a particular plant belongs to. The family name is capitalized but not italicized.
- **Genus:** A group of related plants within a family. The genus is always written in italics with the first letter capitalized, and refers to the generic name of the plant.
- **Species:** The specific name of the plant. Always written in italics; the first letter is lowercased.
- **Chemotype:** An unusually high content of a particular chemical constituent in a plant within the same species.

Let's use rosemary as an example.

- **Family:** Lamiaceae
- **Genus:** *Rosmarinus*
- **Species:** *officinalis*
- **Chemotype:** camphor, cineole, and verbenone

This is how these chemotypes (abbreviated ct.) are written and what makes them different:

- *Rosmarinus officinalis* ct. camphor is rich in the chemical camphor and works as a diuretic, a muscle relaxant, and an emmenagogic (promotes menstruation).
- *Rosmarinus officinalis* ct. cineole is rich in the chemical 1,8-cineole, which is an exceptional antifungal and anti-inflammatory agent.
- *Rosmarinus officinalis* ct. verbenone is high in the chemicals verbenone and pinene and acts as a reliever of muscle spasms and an expectorant.[12]

Can you see why knowing the genus, species, and chemotype of an essential oil is so important? There you are, an unsuspecting essential oils consumer trying to overcome inflammatory arthritic pain, so you go online and read that a topical solution of rosemary essential oil can help. Being a faithful, safe essential oils user, you remember that your favorite essential oils guru always harped on her readers to make sure that they treat their condition with the correct plant species. You purchase *Rosmarinus officinalis,* but inadvertently get a bottle filled with the camphor chemotype, not the cineole variety. Not only does your pain remain, you fear that it's gotten worse and your monthly cycle gets out of whack because you're taking an emmenagogue!

It's important to note that the chemotype doesn't indicate the most prominent chemical in the oil. Rather, it shows which one or two components are drastically elevated. For example, the main chemical in *Rosmarinus* ct. verbenone is still 1,8-cineole.

To complicate matters even more, biochemist Nacim Zouari, PhD, points out, "In the literature and in most cases, only the main constituents of essential oils have been considered for the chemotype's determination. However, it is worth noting that minor compounds can play a very important role in the chemical polymorphism of a given species. In addition, the biological activity of an essential oil may be due to a synergistic action of some minor compounds. In this way, an essential oil is defined not only by its major compounds, but rather by a majority of all its compounds."[13]

During my interview with chemist Dr. Robert Pappas for the Essential Oils Revolution 2 summit, he pointed out that a lack of proper education about the true chemical nature of essential oils is a fundamental problem. This is why I'm going into so much detail about the "sciencey" aspects of essential oils. "Unfortunately, [the average person doesn't] understand the synergistic nature of essential oils, how complex the mixtures are, and how complicated they are, with hundreds and hundreds of molecules in one essential oil," Pappas said. "There are so many interactions that are going on. You can't just say, 'Let's look at pure menthol. And we have this data that says it's this. And because the pure menthol acts this way, well, therefore peppermint must be the same.' You can't do that."[14]

So what's the bottom line?

1. Read the labels.
2. The recipes in this book do not require you to seek out specific chemotypes. However, realize that the plant species doesn't always guarantee the therapeutic nature of the oil due to the chemical anomalies that can occur. This is where chemotypes, indicated by "ct." on the label, come in. As you become more advanced in your study of essential oils and prepare more advanced blends, be sure that you're using the right species and chemotype according to your needs.

There is an entire science devoted to the chemistry and taxonomy of plants and essential oils, which is way beyond the scope of this book. If this topic interests you, check out the additional suggested reading material I've provided in the resource section of this book.

HOW PURE ARE THE ESSENTIAL OILS THAT YOU BUY?

You know what they say: "You don't talk about religion, politics, or your essential oils brand at Thanksgiving dinner!" There is no topic that is more hotly debated in the essential oils world than which company sells the purest oil.

First off, there is no "best," but there are several reputable companies that sell quality oils free of chemical contamination. With that said, Robert Pappas, PhD, told me during our interview for my first telesummit that he estimates more than 75 percent of all the essential oils on the market are adulterated, which means they are either diluted or contaminated with synthetic materials.[15] Essential oil purity and adulteration are extremely important topics when considering which oils to buy. I'll discuss how to choose the right essential oil brands in chapter 2.

Let's debunk two myths about purity in one fell swoop: (1) Purity doesn't guarantee that you'll enjoy a therapeutic effect, and (2) purity doesn't guarantee safety.

If you try an oil and do not get the desired result, it doesn't necessarily mean that the oil is fake or not "pure." It may have more to do with the chemical constituents that are within each batch, which may mean that you'll need to try several different brands to find the one that works for you. And don't believe the "detox" myth. If you apply an essential oil straight (neat) on your skin and experience a rash, bumps, or other adverse effects such as swelling or itching, this does not mean the essential oil is cleansing your body of harmful toxins. Rather, this is known as a "sensitization" response; I'll cover this at length in chapter 2.

MAXIMIZING THE SHELF LIFE OF YOUR ESSENTIAL OILS

You may have heard that essential oils never expire, but don't believe it—essential oils don't last forever. When it comes to storing your essential oils, oxygen is your enemy. More specifically, oxidation (caused by gradual exposure to oxygen) is your enemy because it will cause the the freshness of your oils to plummet and their therapeutic potency to diminish.

The shelf life of most oils ranges from two to four years. It is best to store them in cool, dark places, tightly capped, out of the sun, and away from extreme heat. This is because heat can expedite oxidation, not because heat will destroy the natural characteristics of the compounds in the essential oils. That's another myth.

Two ways to extend the shelf life of your oils beyond two to four years are to store them in the fridge and to mix them with fractionated coconut oil, which doesn't go rancid like other carrier oils.

SAFETY CONSIDERATIONS

Did you know that more than 128,000 people die every year because of adverse reactions to drugs given in the hospital?[16] Just think how high this number would skyrocket if we had data on people dying from drug reactions outside the hospital!

Thankfully, no one is on recent record as dying from essential oils, but to say that they have no side effects is false.[17] However, you'll be relieved to learn that essential oils are at the bottom of the list of substances that cause moderate to serious adverse reactions from overexposure. Statistically, swimming in a pool is more dangerous than using essential oils![18]

Still, safety is the primary focus of most aromatherapists, and for good reason. As much as I love my essential oils, it's important to remember that they do not come without risks. They are still highly concentrated plant-based compounds that should be handled with great care, especially around children.

Just think about it for a minute. As natural as essential oils are, they still need to be extracted using man-made techniques or else they're virtually useless to humans. Fact is, our skin isn't designed to come into contact with neat (undiluted) essential oils for any length of time. They are simply too concentrated and our body cannot process them properly.

I'll instruct you how to use essential oils safely and effectively in upcoming chapters (especially chapter 3), but if you want to learn more about safety, see the additional suggested reading on this subject in the Recommended Resources section.

DECIPHERING THE RESEARCH

As you read this book you'll learn that there are thousands of research studies that discuss the therapeutic use and potential safety concerns of essential oils and their chemical constituents. Primarily because of the money needed to conduct research and the organizations that provide this funding, the medical literature is much more heavily weighted on the constituent side—meaning that a vast majority of the research has been done on individual, isolated chemicals that make up essential oils, and not the oils themselves. These are called "constituent studies" and they are more common because pharmaceutical companies can easily duplicate these isolated chemicals, create synthetic varieties, and include them in their drugs. A prime example is menthol and peppermint. At the time I wrote this book, there were 2,741 published peer-reviewed studies discussing the many aspects of menthol,[19] whereas only 407 addressed peppermint oil specifically.[20]

The significance here lies in the fact that far too many blogs and books offer very detailed advice on how to use oils based on the studies of their chemical components—not of the oils themselves, which is incredibly misleading.

Let's say you're reading a blog post about someone's total remission of chronic migraines after applying diluted peppermint over her temples. Because the essential oil she used was high in menthol, and there are some studies suggesting that menthol can help with migraines,[21] she's now telling everyone with the same condition to use oils rich in menthol (not just peppermint) to get the same result, and her story is being shared all over the Internet.

It is important to note that it is unclear whether the migraines disappeared because of the menthol or because of the cornucopia of chemicals working in synergistic harmony within the peppermint oil. In other words, straight menthol has a different therapeutic effect than peppermint, even though peppermint contains menthol, because there are other chemicals at work in the essential oil.

Furthermore, relying on constituent research can cause people to become overly cautious about the oils that they use. Take, for example, anethole, the primary chemical in star anise and sweet fennel.

Suppose we have an average aromatherapist who teaches about the safe, conservative use of essential oils. This person has a client who is on blood thinners and who took an oral dose of fennel oil, which is believed to prevent blood clots because it contains anethole.[22] Then the client gets injured and has to be rushed to the hospital to tend to his wounds because they won't stop bleeding. Now the aromatherapist is telling everyone taking that same drug never to use anethole-containing essential oils, and this recommendation goes viral in the online community. Again, this is an illogical conclusion because there is no way to determine whether or not the bleeding occurred because of the anethole, the fennel oil as a whole, or because of some outside variable like stress!

The take-home message here is twofold.

- First, we already discussed biochemical individuality, so I won't go into that other than to say that this principle goes both ways: It applies to both therapeutic and safety aspects of aromatherapy. Meaning, what may be unsafe for one person may not necessarily be unsafe for another.
- Second, one must make a significant logical leap to extrapolate data from a constituent study (whether it concerns safety or therapeutic aspects) and draw conclusions about essential oils that contain that particular constituent. You'll hear the loudest voices in the industry (aromatherapists, bloggers, and people

who sell essential oils for a living) making misleading claims by concluding that people should or should not do certain things because of information reported in constituent studies, and this is bad science.

FENNEL ACCUSED OF CAUSING CANCER?!?

Robert Pappas and Nacim Zouari aren't alone in their conclusion that we cannot base safety and therapeutic guidelines on research studies that evaluate the primary chemical constituent(s) in essential oils. A brilliant article discussing the potential carcinogenicity of estragole—a chemical component found in fennel essential oil—puts things into perspective.

The article, published in the journal *Evidence-Based Complementary and Alternative Medicine* by Italian researchers in 2012,[23] looks back at a 1983 study that has shaped decades of practitioners' opinions about fennel. This original study showed that estragole, a constituent of fennel essential oil, caused liver cancer in mice that had yet to be weaned,[24] causing fennel to develop a reputation as a carcinogen. You can understand that no practitioner would want to recommend an essential oil that could potentially cause cancer, right? I know I can. But the study didn't evaluate fennel essential oil—it looked only at its *constituent*. So does that mean fennel essential oil should be banned forever?

The Italian researchers cautioned against making conclusions about essential oils based on constituent studies. "This allegation do[es] not consider [that] the remedy is prepared as a matrix of substances," they said, "and recent researches confirm that pure estragole is inactivated by many substance [sic] contained in the decoction [the liquid that results from boiling or heating plants in water]."

Isolated estragole has become a concern for some researchers, despite fennel's long history of being used medicinally in the following ways:

• Fennel oil has been used widely as a flavoring agent in a variety of foods, as well as in pharmaceutical and cosmetic products.

- Fennel infusions are the classical decoction for nursing babies to prevent flatulence and colic spasm.
- Fennel powder is used as a poultice for snakebites.
- The whole fennel herb has traditionally been heralded in Europe and Mediterranean areas for its ability to act as an analgesic, anti-inflammatory, antioxidant, antispasmodic, diuretic, and galactagogue (promotes lactation).

Conducting a complete literature review, the Italian researchers discovered that all of the animal studies reviewed showing potential estragole toxicity referred to isolated, purified estragole. Thus, the findings gave a toxicological profile only of this one molecule and not the extremely complex phytochemical matrix that makes up fennel essential oil.

Again, it is not sound science to make premature conclusions regarding the safety and risk of a plant or the essential oil extracted from said plant based on constituent studies.[25] Nonetheless, you'll see arbitrary lists on well-known blogs reporting that fennel oil is potentially carcinogenic and should be avoided in people with cancer.[26]

What a shame . . .

This is why I try not to make firm conclusions about which essential oils are best for specific conditions, or which ones to avoid, unless there is definitive research on the entire oil and not just one chemical constituent. Please keep this in mind as I report what the research says about how to use essential oils safely and effectively. I do my best to present a well-balanced approach to safety and therapeutic efficacy and my end goal is to help you find your way through the maze that confuses so many people online.

When I present a list of oils that *could* work to reach a desired health outcome, I do so to show that there are options and to steer you in the right direction. But there is no guarantee that any of those listed will accomplish the desired goal. Remember, we all have different biochemical makeups. Essentially, I'm giving you a fishing pole—to help you figure out what will work for you—and not the fish.

2

Basic Tools and Techniques

Give a man a fish and you feed him for a day; teach a man to fish and you feed him for a lifetime.

—*MAIMONIDES*

My mission in writing this book is not to give you a fish, but to give you a fishing pole that you can use to regain control of your health. As a biblical health educator, I'm passionate about making that fishing pole the best, most useful tool it can be—and about empowering you to know where, when, and how to use it.

In chapter 1 I covered the fundamentals of aromatherapy, which includes history, extraction methods, different aromatic products, taxonomy, and general safety considerations.

In this chapter, I want to cover the fundamentals of how to incorporate essential oils safely and effectively into your natural health regimen, the tools that you'll need, and tips on how to use them.

STOCKING YOUR TOOLBOX: ESSENTIAL OILS, CARRIER OILS, DIFFUSERS, AND CONTAINERS

If I were a master craftsman (which I am not!), I could tell you how to build a house, but if you didn't have the materials you wouldn't get too far. Right? Same thing here.

Before you can get started on your journey to master the art and practice of essential oils, you need the right tools.

I promise to keep the list short and the items affordable so that you don't get too hung up on this phase. I want you to be able to get started as quickly and painlessly as possible; but I also want you to experience noticeable benefits—and if you grab a random, nontherapeutic-grade bottle of tea tree oil off the drugstore shelf and start dabbing it on your athlete's foot (which is exactly what I did once, many years ago), either nothing will happen or your skin will get irritated, and you will decide that all this essential oil talk is just that—talk.

You can easily find all of the aromatherapy supplies for these recipes on Amazon. They are readily available and cost-effective. Please note that I don't recommend specific brands, but I do include a detailed guide on how to choose the right brand(s) later in this chapter.

TOOL #1: ESSENTIAL OILS

You can purchase essential oils from several sources, including online vendors, health food stores, and natural grocery stores. I like patronizing specialty, locally owned apothecaries, as the staff who work there are often well-versed in the criteria the store uses to select the brands they carry. Some yoga studios and chiropractors also sell them.

Be very careful about what you buy at national chain stores. If an oil is labeled 100 percent pure and is being sold at a dirt-cheap price, it's probably too good to be true. For example, the lavender essential oil sold at one national chain has been proven to be adulterated with large amounts of synthetic linalool and synthetic linalyl acetate.[1]

Be especially careful when reading labels. With essential oils, there is nothing on the label that you can truly trust other than plant taxonomy, plant sourcing, extraction method, and chemotype. Everything else is marketing propaganda. The prime example is the all-too-common "therapeutic grade" claim that you'll read on many labels, which is intended to imply that the oils are of a superior quality compared to nontherapeutic-grade oils. Not to burst anyone's bubble, but this is a marketing strategy and doesn't mean much at all, because all essential oils are therapeutic if they are pure! Contaminated essential oils really aren't essential oils at all, but a combination of synthetic chemicals, some essential oils components, and God only knows what else.

Three facts to keep in mind:

1. Many companies have developed internal therapeutic-grade standards, which essentially boil down to purity. Meaning, any reputable company will have its oils tested by multiple third parties to guarantee that they are not adulterated with synthetic chemicals, fillers, or other agents. If the company can prove this, it can most likely be trusted as a viable resource for a good-quality product. Whether it "certifies" this process or calls it a fancy name really doesn't matter.

2. That said, non-adulteration doesn't guarantee therapeutic effectiveness—that depends on the chemical constituency. All purity refers to is whether or not the oil is adulterated with carrier oils or synthetic chemical components.

3. As for supplements and most things in the natural health space, there are no independent governing third-party agencies evaluating and certifying essential oils as "therapeutic" or "pure." What you see on your labels is (hopefully) based on internal testing and standards that each company commits to uphold.

   Many companies pay third parties to evaluate their products and test them for purity, but there is no FDA equivalent in the natural health world. When your favorite brand pays for its oils to be tested by a third party, no one is forcing the company to make sure that its labeling is 100 percent accurate or that it is selling a pure, high-quality oil. Mind you, a "pure" oil can be incorrectly distilled or harvested from a cheaper species that does not contain the volatile organic compounds that a more expensive species or chemotype would contain.

With that information in mind, here is how to choose a reputable oil brand:

1. **Get a referral.** Ask friends and family members whom you respect for a list of their favorite brands. Just be careful to not let multilevel marketing propaganda get in the way of truth. Everyone's favorite brand is the best, right? Especially when that person is selling it!

2. **Find out about sourcing.** Contact the company that you're interested in via email or phone for a report of their sourcing and quality standards.

3. **Get a batch report.** Ask the company for a gas chromatography/mass spectrometry (GC/MS) report of a few oils that you're interested in. These linear graphs are used to identify adulteration and to break down the chemical components of individual oils. This can help you determine the chemotype and potential therapeutic benefits as well as safety issues for that particular oil.

4. **Sample some.** Try a couple of different brands and test for yourself. Lemon, lavender, and peppermint are common, relatively inexpensive oils that should be a good gauge to see if this brand is for you. Notice how your body responds when you smell, feel, and taste the oil. If you get a headache immediately after opening a bottle of peppermint from a particular brand, it doesn't mean that the oil is junk. Maybe the chemicals in the oil come from a chemotype or species that was harvested at a particular time that doesn't respond well to your body. This is why you cannot rest on your laurels and must do an organoleptic evaluation (how your body perceives the oil through the six senses: taste, touch, smell, sight, hearing, and intuition) every time you get a new oil just in case the constituents in the oil don't jibe with your body's chemistry.

Keep in mind that many of the small companies get their oils from the same suppliers. They just use private labels. From what I've been told, the larger companies have unique suppliers, which differentiates their product from their competitors'. This doesn't guarantee purity, but it can help put your mind to rest that they are likely proprietary.

Contamination Concerns

Is organic important? Not necessarily. Like our tainted air, food, and water supply, it is becoming increasingly difficult to find anything free of pesticide residues and toxic contaminants.

In 2014, scientists and essential oil producers met at the International Federation of Essential Oil and Aroma Trades Conference in Rome, Italy, to share their concerns about the quality and safety of our global essential oil supply. These are some of the key takeaways as shared by the founder, president, CEO, and principal of the American College of Healthcare Sciences, Dorene Petersen:[2]

- Unfortunately, essential oils—even those certified as organic—can contain pesticide residues.
- Passive contamination can occur even though a farmer does not actively use pesticides because of "acts of nature" such as wind drift or water runoff from a neighboring field, and from incorrect essential oil storage.
- Pesticides easily dissolve in fats and lipids, making the transition to the essential oil possible.
- Cold-pressed citrus oils are more likely to contain pesticide residues than steam-distilled citrus because pesticides tend to be hydrophilic, thermostable, and volatile.

To check for quality, try answering these questions:

- Does the company have a relationship with its distillers?
- Can the company readily supply a batch-specific GC/MS report on the oil it sells?
- Can the company readily provide material safety data sheets (MSDS) upon request?
- What is the common name, Latin name (genus and species), country of origin, part of plant processed, and type of extraction (distillation or expression), and how was it grown (organic or indigenously sourced)?

In my opinion, one of the most important factors is whether or not the oils are indigenously sourced. Meaning, are they harvested from native plants? This is important because native plants contain essential oils that act as natural insecticides to the pests in that particular area, so growers do not need to use as many chemicals as they do on nonnative plants, which don't have these natural defense mechanisms. Even more important is the fact that nonnative plants pale in comparison to native plants in terms of nutrition and chemical constituency.

My father-in-law is a retired PhD agricultural scientist who spent his career evaluating the chemical compounds in plants. He told me that native plants *always* have a better nutritional and more therapeutic chemical profile because they have evolved to thrive in that specific climate with the particular blend of nutrients found in the soil there.

Indigenous plants:

- Evolved over a long period of time to thrive in their native region.
- Adapted to the local weather and geology.
- Can thrive in drought and inclement weather situations.
- Are environmentally sustainable for pesticide-free farming because they have developed natural resistance to native predators.
- Have a positive impact on the local environment and ecosystem by forming natural "communities" with other plants.

Nonindigenous plants, on the other hand:

- Did not evolve but were unnaturally introduced (deliberately or by accident) into an environment.
- Are not well suited for pesticide-free farming because they are not naturally resistant to native predators.
- Have a negative impact on the local environment and ecosystem because they have a tendency to take over a habitat, require pesticides to thrive, and are not natural food sources for neighboring wildlife.

In short, do the best you can to find the highest-quality oils. Ultimately, though, the proof will be in how the essential oils work for you. If you try an oil and don't notice any benefits, or experience only adverse reactions, it's time to try a different brand before you write off that oil entirely.

TOOL #2: CARRIER OILS

To watch my 3-part video series that covers carrier oils, dilution guides, and tips on roller bottle blends, go to thehealingpowerofessentialoils.com.

Trust me, friends don't let friends use essential oils directly on their skin undiluted (called a "neat" application). It's simply not needed, nor is it safe.

Many essential oils are so concentrated and powerful that you need to dilute them in order to use them effectively. You do this by mixing a few drops of the essential oil with what's known as a carrier oil—a fatty extract of a nut or seed. It might seem backwards to say that diluting a substance makes it more effective, but in this case it is true. If you apply essential oil neat, a few things may happen:

- **You can irritate your skin.** Your skin may be sensitive to the concentrated oil, thwarting the healing benefits that you are seeking to create.
- **You can permanently hurt yourself.** Worse yet, you may become *sensitized* to that particular oil if you don't dilute it with a carrier. A type of allergic response, sensitization may prevent you from ever using that oil again. You'll know if this happens because you'll experience a number of signs and symptoms every time you use a particular oil: headaches, itching, hives, nausea, or a number of other adverse reactions.
- **You'll waste money.** Being volatile, essential oils will quickly evaporate off the surface of your skin, whereas the fats in the carrier can help prevent this and ensure that the essential oils will penetrate into your pores.
- **It's not sustainable.** As essential oil demand skyrockets, we will most certainly see a growing list of endangered and extinct plants unless we change our ways. By diluting in a carrier, you're using less essential oil while getting

the same therapeutic effect without the safety risks. Not to mention, you're doing your part to help make sure our babies and grandbabies can enjoy these wonderful gifts from nature that we all too often take for granted. It's a win-win-win!

While there are some rare instances when neat is desirable—gentle oils, or oils used under the supervision of a trained professional—your best bet is to dilute essential oils in a carrier every time (see the Roller Bottle Dilution Guide in chapter 7 for more information on how to do this).

Once you get the hang of it, adding your essential oils to a carrier first is hardly any extra work. I'll walk you through the more common carrier oils, but if you run into one that isn't covered here, take the time to look it up and learn what it is and what it does.

1. Beginner Carrier Oils: Olive and Coconut

- **Olive oil.** Extra-virgin olive oil is the ideal, because it is cold pressed (not extracted using high heat or harsh chemicals) and minimally processed. It has a light green color and a heavy scent. As with essential oils, olive oil adulteration is a huge concern. Test yours at home to make sure it's not cut with any fillers or cheaper oils: Pure olive oil will harden in the fridge.
- **Coconut oil.** A saturated fat extracted from coconuts, this luscious oil penetrates the skin easily with very little greasy residue, conveying the oils you've blended in.
- **Fractionated coconut oil.** Literally a fraction of the coconut oil (all of the long-chain fatty acids have been removed via hydrolysis and steam distillation so that the oil stays liquid at room temperature, unlike standard coconut oil), fractionated coconut oil is a lightweight emollient that is a must-have for dry or sensitive skin. It is considered to be the most cost-effective oil because it will never go rancid, and helps preserve the shelf life of your essential oils when blended.

2. Intermediate Carrier Oils: Almond and Jojoba

- **Almond oil.** Very mild in scent and flavor, almond oil is nutrient dense and versatile.
- **Jojoba oil.** Pronounced *ho-HO-ba*, jojoba has a thicker consistency that's well suited to deep penetration. Jojoba has an excellent shelf life, which makes it perfect for storing until you need it for small dilution preparations.

3. Advanced Carrier Oils

These fruit-seed oils are as edible as the other options we've covered so far. These choices may cost a little more, but are relatively easy to find. They are readily available on Amazon and at your local health food store.

- **Apricot oil.** Apricot oil is available as expeller pressed or cold pressed; the only difference between the two forms is simply texture so you can let preference and availability be your guide in choosing between them.
- **Avocado oil.** Avocado oil is taken from the smooth flesh around the pit.
- **Grapeseed oil.** Also a culinary oil, grapeseed oil is a carrier oil with a light texture and lack of residue.
- **Borage oil.** Taken from the seeds of a flowering perennial herb, borage oil is often consumed for its gamma linolenic acid (GLA) content.
- **Evening primrose oil.** Named for flowers that open only in the evenings, evening primrose oil is a more delicate oil that must be cold pressed and should be refrigerated. It is used in culinary preparations as well as many women's health blends.

My Go-To Carrier Oil Blend

Most DIY recipes call for a carrier oil in one form or another. You can usually choose the one you like best unless a recipe calls for something specific.

In our house, we like to use a combination of carrier oils that my wife devised when she was pregnant with our first child, Esther, to hydrate her skin and prevent stretch marks. She combined her favorite ingredients based on their benefits:

- Unrefined, organic coconut oil for its antifungal and antibacterial properties
- Sweet almond oil because it's great for skin health and won't mask the aroma of the essential oils you'll add
- Jojoba oil because it penetrates the skin so well
- Vitamin E for its antioxidant-rich, skin-repairing ability

Mama Z has had four babies so far and you'd never guess it by looking at her tummy! She's fit and toned, and she credits her glowing (stretch-mark-free!) skin to this oil base she created nearly ten years ago.

In the recipes that are scattered throughout this book, I often suggest this blend as a base for its versatility and its healing powers in its own right. (You might want to put a sticky note on this page, so you can easily refer back to it—until you've made it so many times that you've memorized the recipe!)

MAMA Z'S OIL BASE

We use this for everything in our home! It's great to always have on hand and will meet most of your DIY needs.

54 ounces raw organic, unrefined coconut oil (melted)
16 ounces sweet almond oil
8 ounces jojoba oil
4 ounces vitamin E

SUPPLIES
Quart or pint wide-mouth mason jars

1. If you're in a colder climate and need to liquefy your coconut oil, be sure to preserve the nutrition content by using indirect heat to warm it up instead of heating it on the stove. We have placed a glass measuring cup with coconut oil in it on a space heater or the top of our gas stove while we're baking something in the oven to slowly melt the oil. You can also immerse a jar of coconut oil in a bowl or saucepan of warm (not boiling) water for a few minutes until the oil liquefies.

2. Combine all of the ingredients in a large cooking pot and mix using a wire whisk or a blender to reach a smoother, "whipped" consistency if desired.

3. Pour into quart or pint mason jars or other glass containers. Store in a cool, dark place, where it will last for 1 to 2 years.

Notes: *Once your base oil is ready, you can make your own blends; use 6 to 12 drops of essential oils for every 1 ounce of the base.*

This recipe makes a lot—it really is that versatile and can be used to formulate multiple healing salves and balms (that also make great gifts). Be sure to store any oil base that you aren't using right away out of sunlight—the saturated fats in coconut milk won't spoil, but the almond oil could get stale. You can also easily divide the recipe by a quarter to make a smaller batch.

Depending on the temperature in your house, the base may go back to a solid or semisolid state (coconut oil has a melting point of 76 degrees). If it hardens, you can either liquefy some by rubbing it in your hands, placing it near a heating vent, or putting it near the oven when you're cooking dinner.

➡ To watch me and Mama Z make her oil base and to learn more about carrier oils, go to HealingPowerOfEssentialOils.com and click on the "Demo Videos" tab.

Why You Should Use Glass

In this recipe and many of the recipes to come, you'll notice that I often call for glass bowls and bottles for mixing and storing essential oil–based products. Here's why:

- Essential oils have a tendency to break down the petrochemicals in plastic, which can cause carcinogens and other dangerous chemicals to leach out into your home remedies.
- Similarly, it's a good idea to avoid aluminum and stainless steel containers, as essential oils can cause the heavy metals in these materials to leach out into your blends.

The one category where using a glass storage container is a concern is for products you will use in the shower or bathtub. Since tile shower floors and bathtubs are often slippery, it's easy to slip and drop a bottle. If you are concerned that this may happen, you can store your shampoos, conditioners, and body scrubs in PET (polyethylene terephthalate) plastic as it does not contain known hormone disruptors such as bisphenol-A and is easily recyclable (it is labeled with the number 1 inside the recycling symbol that typically appears on the bottom of plastic containers).

TOOL #3: EMULSIFIERS, PRESERVATIVES, AND SOLUBILIZERS

If you plan on having some DIY fun, you'll want to have some natural preservatives and emulsifiers on hand. In a nutshell:

- Emulsifiers contain a hydrophilic head and a hydrophobic tail that help essential oils and water mix together to create emulsions. An emulsion is a seamless blend of two fluids that normally don't mix, such as oil and water; lotions, creams, and even mayonnaise are examples of emulsions. Otherwise, your essential oils will float on top of your water-based DIY cleaning and body care solutions, which is not only inefficient but also a safety hazard. Examples of emulsifiers include aloe vera oil (not gel), castile soap, emulsifying wax, lecithin, organic grain alcohol (190 proof), and vitamin E TPGS (a water-soluble derivative of vitamin E).
- Preservatives help maintain the shelf life and therapeutic efficacy of water-based products that have a tendency to go rancid or develop bacterial overgrowth if not treated. Examples of conventional preservatives include potentially harmful chemicals like Liquid Germall Plus and Optiphen. These chemicals contain propylene glycol—a known skin irritant used to make polyester compounds and artificial smoke/fog for firefighter training and theater performances.[3] Unfortunately, I am unfamiliar with any preservatives that are safe and actually work for the everyday DIY enthusiast.
- Solubilizers will help a solute dissolve into a solvent, which means they will literally help dissolve oil in water. Imagine drawing a nice bath at the end of

the night to help you decompress after a long day at work. If you don't solubilize the essential oils that you add to your bath, they end up floating in little isolated bubbles on top of the water—and when you sit in the tub, you may end up exposing your genitals to fully concentrated essential oils. Examples of solubilizers include solubol and polysorbate 20, which I'm not a big fan of because it can become contaminated with 1,4-dioxane, a known animal carcinogen that penetrates readily into the skin. Solubol is the best natural choice, but can be difficult to purchase if you don't know where to get less common aromatherapy supplies.

Factions of the aromatherapy community are somewhat at odds with one another about balancing the convenience and safety of using chemical-based emulsifiers, preservatives, and solubilizers against the obvious safety concerns of microbial contamination, rancidity, and inadvertent application of neat oils to the skin.

Something just doesn't sit right with me about using chemicals in essential oil–based products—it seems to defeat the purpose of using essential oils to begin with (seeing as we're trying to avoid exposure to potentially toxic chemicals in our body care and home products).

So what is the solution? Regarding preservatives, be sure to use up your water-based formulations (such as spritzers and sprays) within a couple of weeks, and consider refrigerating them. Also use distilled (sterile) water when possible to reduce bacteria growth. (Note: Since hydrosols tend to become rancid fairly quickly and can be easily tainted by microbial overgrowth, I've chosen not to include recipes for them in this book.) To learn more about hydrosols, check out the good aromatherapy reference texts in the Recommended Resources section at the end of this book.

Finding safe emulsifiers and solubilizers is not as troublesome because they are readily available online. You really can't avoid them in your spritzers, hand sanitizers, and other water-based products or else you'll spray straight essential oils into the air and onto your skin, which is wasteful and dangerous. Personally, I have found that aloe vera oil, castile soap, and organic grain alcohol are the best all-around solutions for my needs.

TOOL #4: DIFFUSER

An ultrasonic diffuser is a small machine, similar to a humidifier, that breaks essential oils down into minuscule components and then disperses them through the air, carrying tiny doses of the oil directly throughout the room and ultimately into your respiratory system. My wife and I have diffusers running at various times throughout the day and use them at night to help us get a better night's sleep—they enhance our mood and our health, and the mood and health of our kids, too!

In addition, diffusing essential oils benefits your health and saves you money by allowing you to throw away those scented plug-ins and air fresheners, which emit toxic chemicals that have been linked to cardiac dysfunction, migraines, neurotoxicity, and cancer.[4]

For all these reasons, I believe every house should have a diffuser in every room. Even the nursery! Not only will they help make your house smell and feel refreshing, but they also emit aromatic "volatiles" that have significant medicinal properties. With an average cost of around $50 for a diffuser (or much less for one you can fashion yourself out of things that you already have on hand), that's a good cost-benefit ratio. Thanks to the booming popularity of essential oils, there are nearly as many different diffusers as there are oils: ultrasonic or humidifying; heat diffusers; nebulizers; reed diffusers; USB car diffusers—and many others. My preference is the ultrasonic variety. They are simple to use and are easy to clean. Just simply wipe the container with a dry cloth or paper towel. They are also extremely effective at dispersing essential oils throughout rooms as large as 1000 square feet and come in a plethora of stylish designs.

Quick Blending Tips

I recommend premixing blends and storing them in 5 ml essential oil bottles, which you can easily get on Amazon or at your local health food store. Then you add anywhere from 2 drops (average-sized car diffuser) to 25 drops (average-sized nebulizer) of these blends in total.

A few tips on blending—no recipe required!:

- Start by making a small quantity (10 drops in total max) so you don't waste much if you don't like the blend.
- The chemistry (efficacy) of the blend is not impacted by the order in which you pour your oils.
- Start off by using the following ratio: 25% top notes; 50% middle notes; 25% base notes. See "Follow Your Nose" for more details.
- Using glass pipettes helps minimize spills—having a few on hand makes formulating your own blends very convenient.
- Absolutes go a long way. You only need a drop or two per blend.
- Remember to write down formulas you like so you can remember your ratios for next time!

Follow Your Nose

When blending essential oils, it's a good idea to take guidance from traditional perfumery by following what's known as "aromatic note classifications." These classifications designate how scents are perceived once they are applied to the body. In a nutshell:

- **Top/head notes** are the first impression of any blend, evaporate quickly and are quick to dissipate. They are usually described as "light" and "sharp." Common essential oils with top/head notes include eucalyptus, lemon, and peppermint.
- **Middle/heart notes** are experienced next and supply the dominant aroma of the blend. Classic examples include clary sage, neroli, and ylang ylang.
- **Base/bottom notes** are the foundation of the blend. Known to be heavy, dense, and strong, common examples include frankincense, patchouli, and vetiver.

AROMATIC NOTE CLASSIFICATION

TOP NOTES	MIDDLE NOTES	BASS NOTES
Anise	Bay	Angelica Root
Basil	Cajuput	Balsam, Peru
Bay Laurel	Carrot Seed	Beeswax
Bergamot	Chamomile, German	Benzoin
Bergamot Mint	Chamomile, Roman	Cedarwood
Citronella	Cinnamon	Frankincense
Eucalyptus	Clary Sage	Ginger
Galbanum	Clove Bud	Helichrysum
Grapefruit	Cypress	Myrrh
Lavender	Dill	Oakmoss
Lavandin	Elemi	Olibanum
Lemon	Fennel	Patchouli
Lemongrass	Fir Needle	Sandalwood
Lime	Geranium	Vanilla
Orange	Hyssop	Vetiver
Peppermint	Jasmine	
Petitgrain	Juniper Berry	
Spearmint	Linden Blossom	
Tangerine	Marjoram	
	Neroli	
	Nutmeg	
	Palmarosa	
	Parsley	
	Pepper, Black	
	Pine, Scotch	
	Rose	
	Rose Geranium	
	Rosemary	
	Rosewood	
	Spruce	
	Tea Tree	
	Thyme	
	Yarrow	
	Ylang Ylang	

From "Aromatic Blending of Essential Oils," AromaWeb.com.

Diffuser Blends

In accordance with the blending tips and aromatic note classification I just shared, here are some nice blends that Mama Z and I like to make. We switch ours up depending on our mood and the season.

- **Holiday Blend:** Fir needle (Balsam fir, Douglas fir, white fir), peppermint, and vanilla absolute
- **Deep Breathing Blend:** Cardamom, eucalyptus, lemon, peppermint, rosemary, and tea tree
- **Focus Blend:** Cedarwood, frankincense, sandalwood, and vetiver
- **Good-Bye Allergy Blend:** Lavender, lemon, and peppermint
- **Healthy Digestion Blend:** Anise, caraway, fennel, ginger, lemon, and tarragon
- **Modern-Day Anointing Blend:** Cassia, cinnamon leaf, frankincense, and myrrh
- **Immunity-Boosting Blend:** Cinnamon bark, cinnamon leaf, clove, frankincense, rosemary, orange, and lemon
- **Joyful Blend:** Orange, lemon, bergamot, grapefruit, and vanilla absolute
- **Sleepy-Time Blend:** Roman chamomile, lavender, and vetiver

TOOL #5: INHALERS AND OTHER DIY SUPPLIES

Because essential oils need to be diluted for many preparations, you'll want containers to store your blends—and several of each type of container. If you already have some in your medicine cabinet, be sure to clean them in the dishwasher and allow them to dry completely before refilling with your healing essential oil blends.

- 1-, 2-, and 4-ounce dark glass bottles with screw tops—the darkness of the glass prevents the oils from oxidizing due to or being damaged by exposure to light. *Best for:* Massage oil blends.
- 1-, 2-, 4-, 16-, and 32-ounce glass with spray tops. *Best for:* Spritzes, such

as air fresheners, spot removers, hair spray, hand sanitizers, and household cleaners.

- 5, 10, and 15 ml dark glass bottles with roller tops. *Best for:* Travel, or for applying rubs or massage oils to wriggly kids.
- A couple of aromatherapy inhaler tubes—plastic, lip balm–sized tubes with tight-fitting caps that make it easy to take a whiff of a custom blend.

Techniques: Inhalation, Topical Application, Internal Use, Cooking, Oil Pulling

By this point, you should have at least a few essential oils on hand, as well as carrier oil, containers, and perhaps a diffuser. In this section, you'll learn a number of key techniques that will help you develop your own essential oils practice that you can customize to your needs and continually refine over time. All right, you've got your gear. Now here's a little Fishing 101.

Inhalation

Two of the most effective and popular ways to utilize aromatherapy are diffusers and personal inhalers. Because steam diffusion breaks up the volatile organic compounds and disperses them into millions of microparticles, oils diffused throughout a room are relatively safe for most people.

To enjoy the aromatic benefits of essential oils via diffusion, simply:

- Fill your diffuser with tap water up to the "fill line" or fill marker (or simmer a pot of water on the stove).
- Use 4 or 5 drops of essential oil per 100–150 ml water (the amount depends on your diffuser's water capacity). For inhaled oils, you need only a small amount to create a big impact.

That's it! The benefits last after the diffusion has ended; there is no need to run the diffuser continuously unless you prefer it.

Safety Tips: Always use diffusers in a well-ventilated room, especially if you have children or pets. When you're starting out, or when you're using a new blend, diffuse oils for just few minutes to give your body a "taste" of what's in there. If you don't have any adverse reactions (headaches, sinus issues, etc.), then gradually work your way up to running your diffuser for a few hours at a time.

To use an inhaler, simply place a precut organic cotton pad inside your inhaler tube and add drops of your desired essential oils directly to the cotton pad. Look for cotton pads that are specifically designed for use in aromatherapy inhalers (you can find these on Amazon.com). Once created, your inhaler can last up to one year, depending on how often you open it up and use it; the more you open the lid, the more oxygen the essential oils are exposed to, and the more quickly they will oxidize and evaporate.

Topical Application

Applying essential oils onto your skin (most often diluted in a carrier oil) is the second most common way to access their healing powers. As I've explained, dilution is not only wise, it's also necessary to ensure safety and efficacy. Depending on what you're trying to accomplish, it is generally advised that you dilute as follows:

- 0.5%–1%: For children, the face, and sensitive skin like genitals and underarms.
- 2%: Standard adult dilution for most DIY applications.
- 3%–5%: For chronic conditions like aches and pains.
- 5%–10%: For acute conditions like burns and cuts and for specifically treating a disease for up to one week at a time.
- 10%+: To be used with great care and only for a very short period of time.
- 25%+: To be used only under the supervision of a trained health care provider.

Here's a quick guide to knowing how many drops of essential oil to add:

	% DILUTION	EO DROPS PER OUNCE	EO DROPS PER TABLESPOON
Infants and children	0.5%	3	1.5
	1.0%	6	3
Adults	2.0%	12	6
	3.0%	18	9
	5.0%	30	15
	10.0%	60	30

Note: There are 2 tablespoons in 1 ounce. Mix the essential oil with the carrier, then apply as indicated by the recipe or remedy for that particular ailment. You've now successfully diluted your essential oil and enjoyed the added benefit of a nourishing carrier oil.

WHERE TO APPLY YOUR DILUTED ESSENTIAL OILS

You may have heard that applying essential oils to the bottom of your feet is the most effective way to get the healing compounds into your bloodstream. This is not actually true. Research has determined that this is the order of areas of the body where the skin is most permeable, from highest to lowest:[5]

1. Genital region
2. Head and neck region
3. Trunk (chest, stomach, back)
4. Arms (including the hands and fingers)
5. Legs (including the bottom of the feet)

This doesn't mean you should apply essential oils to your genitals! In fact, the researchers who published this paper recommend: "Transdermal formulations should be applied to the trunk or the arm as there is usually less potential for sensitization and the lower density of hair follicles leads to better tack and ease of removal." It also means that applying essential oils to the soles of your feet is, contrary to popular belief, the least effective (not to mention slipperiest!) way to get essential oils into your bloodstream via the skin.

Safety Tip: Before putting a new oil or blend on your skin, do a skin patch test by applying a 1% dilution on the back of your hand or the bottom of your foot—this is the same concept as testing carpet cleaner on an inconspicuous spot first before potentially staining a large area. Let the mixture settle for a few minutes and observe. If you experience no adverse reactions (bumps, burns, rashes, etc.) within ten minutes, this is a good sign that you can gradually scale up to more concentrated dilutions.

THE PERILS OF PHOTOSENSITIZATION

Some essential oils can increase the photosensitivity of your skin. For example, chemicals in the citrus family such as *bergapten* are notable for their phototoxic effects. When bergapten is left on the skin and then exposed to the sun, it can amplify the effect of UV rays, potentially causing sunburn and leading to sun spots. Some people just decide not to use any bergapten-heavy oils topically, but simply avoiding the sun after use (for example, by applying them at night) is sufficient. Alternatively, use steam-distilled citrus oils, which have lower concentrations of bergapten and mitigate this effect.

PHOTOSENSITIZERS

ESSENTIAL OIL	LATIN NAME
Angelica root	*Angelica archangelica*
Bergamot	*Citrus bergamia*
Bitter orange, expressed	*Citrus aurantium*
Cumin	*Cuminum cyminum*
Grapefruit	*Citrus paradisi*
Lemon, expressed	*Citrus limon*
Lime, expressed	*Citrus medica*
Rue	*Ruta graveolens*

NONPHOTOTOXIC CITRUS OILS

ESSENTIAL OIL	LATIN NAME
Bergamot: Bergaptenless (FCF: Furanocoumarin Free)	*Citrus bergamia*
Lemon, distilled	*Citrus limon*
Lime, distilled	*Citrus medica*
Mandarin	*Citrus reticulata*
Sweet or wild orange	*Citrus sinensis*
Tangelo	*Citrus tangelo*
Tangerine, expressed	*Citrus reticulata*
Yuzu oil	*Citrus juno*

From Tisserand and Young's *Essential Oil Safety.*[6]

Great care should be taken when using citrus oils during summer months and with your children in general, but you don't have to avoid them altogether. Many aromatherapists agree that heavily diluting citrus oils minimizes the risk.

Considerations for Consuming Essential Oils

Some oils are safe for ingestion. A common preparation is to add a few drops to a beverage, such as water, and then drink it, though that's not the best idea unless you use a solubilizer like alcohol or (my favorite) liquid stevia extract. The key is to mix the essential oils and liquid stevia (or another emulsifier) first; then add water, juice, tea, or whatever liquid you desire. Remember that oil and water *do not mix,* so simply adding a drop to water will leave that drop undiluted. Some oils are irritants and all are very strong, so it's best to be safe and dilute the oil with an edible carrier like coconut oil first.

Some aromatherapists claim that oils should never be ingested, and most will suggest that people do so only under the care of trained professionals. However, it is important to realize that people consume essential oils every day without even knowing it. Where do you think your processed foods get their flavor? Virtually anything that is naturally flavored most likely contains essential oils.

Moreover, there are no scientific, evidence-based, anatomical, physiological, or logical reasons to say that essentials oils are unsafe for human consumption. Rest assured that large professional organizations like the National Association for Holistic Aromatherapy (NAHA) support safe, internal use. According to NAHA, "Essential oils may be applied on the skin (dermal application), inhaled, diffused or taken internally. Each of these methods has safety issues which need to be considered."[7]

Additionally, the universally acclaimed text *Essential Oil Safety: A Guide for Health Care Professionals* repeatedly refers to "maximum oral dose" in relation to consuming essential oils safely and effectively.[8]

As with many things, a little goes a long way with essential oils, which is why I propose these tried-and-true tips on taking them internally:

1. Always dilute in an edible carrier oil, whether taking as a culinary preparation or in a capsule.
2. Don't overdo it—limit use to two or three drops at a time, and be sure to wait at least four hours before taking consecutive doses.
3. Listen to your body, and . . .
4. Discontinue use *immediately* if adverse reactions occur.

Safety Tip: Taking essential oils internally can possibly put you at risk of drug interactions if you are also taking prescription medication. Unfortunately, what studies do exist that examine potential drug reactions look at individual chemical constituents—there are virtually no studies that evaluate how human patients respond to taking drugs and essential oils together. Yet, as we've already seen, it is not sound science to make definitive claims based on one chemical, because an essential oil can contain dozens if not hundreds of chemicals. That said, it's better to be safe than sorry, especially if you're new to essential oils, so it would be wise to consult with your health care provider before ingesting essential oils if you're taking pharmaceutical or over-the-counter drugs.

Spice Up Your Cooking with Essential Oils

Combining nutritious foods with flavorful spices and herbs is a time-honored tradition. The flowers and herbs that grace our gardens are also delicious sources of wellness. Extending this celebration to cooking with essential oils widens our appreciation for their amazing diversity and abundance and all of the goodness available at our fingertips.

My family and I enjoy using essential oils in our food for a number of reasons:

1. **They make eating more enjoyable.** Essential oils create an invigorating eating experience with their powerful, uplifting aromas.

2. **They restore flavor.** Because modern farming practices have depleted nutrient levels in soil, and because so much produce now travels thousands of miles between the time it's picked and when you buy it at the store, many fresh foods don't taste the way they used to. Those of you who are old enough to remember what fruits and veggies once tasted like understand the difference. Cooking with essential oils brings back that flavor burst!

3. **They're more economical.** What's cheaper, purchasing a $3 organic lemon to zest for your meringue or using a couple drops of lemon oil? One drop of essential oil is the flavor equivalent of about one teaspoon of your average dried herb. Essential oils also have a shelf life that is two to three times longer than dried herbs.

4. **They're easier than herbs.** It's much less time consuming to simply open a bottle and pour in one or two drops of an essential oil than to wash and chop fresh herbs—and there's no knife or cutting board to wash either.

5. **They enhance food safety.** In addition to flavor, essential oils are regularly tested by researchers for their potential to improve food safety. Antimicrobial oils, the theory goes, might be able to minimize foodborne illness if manufacturers added them to packaging.

Cooking with essential oils is nothing new. The important thing is to do so safely, appreciating the differences between a whole herb or spice and its essential oil. Not every essential oil is a good choice for cooking. Sometimes the oil doesn't taste quite as yummy as the whole herb. Sometimes the oil has too much of a certain component, making it less than ideal or even unsafe to ingest in excessive quantities. Fennel is a good example, as when a woman ate an "undisclosed amount" of fennel cakes containing essential oil and wound up having seizures.[9]

The key here is to enjoy essential oils in "culinary dosages," which is generally one to three drops per dish. When we read about cases of "undisclosed amounts" of anything, they're usually extreme amounts that are well beyond the scope of culinary preparations.

Knowing all about the oil you'd like to use—its safety, profile, and precautions—is important. With proper use, cooking with essential oils can be both safe and fun.

Cooking Safely with Essential Oils

- **Reduce.** Remember that the essential oil is a concentrated form of its original source. Just like you use far less cinnamon powder than cinnamon sticks, the essential oil should be used in much smaller quantities than the whole substance. A good rule of thumb is that a drop will replace a teaspoon of the original form, and you don't need more than one or two drops for a full recipe.
- **Dilute.** Another thing to keep in mind when cooking with essential oils is that they should still be diluted in a lipid first. This not only keeps you safe, but also helps to ensure that the oil (and flavor!) gets dispersed throughout the whole dish. For savory recipes, dilute in a bit of olive or coconut oil. Stir, then add to the recipe. For sweet recipes, honey or a syrup works well.
- **Delay.** Finally, for hot foods, wait until the end of cooking before adding the essential oil. They are called "volatile oils" for a reason—they are relatively fragile and will dissipate quickly in high heat. Meaning, if you add the oils too soon, they may evaporate altogether!

  For stovetop recipes, stir your diluted essential oil into the finished dish, after cooking. For baking, you'll simply expect to lose a bit of the flavor and beneficial properties in the process. Dilution throughout the recipe will help, and you'll still be able to enjoy the flavors no matter what!

Use just a drop or two in recipes sweet or savory, cooked or raw. Fewer drops per recipe help to promote good safety for a wide range of oils.

The Magic of Oil Pulling with Essential Oils

Let me share with you an ancient Ayurvedic technique for health that Indians have used for thousands of years to treat dozens of conditions and diseases, ranging from headaches and tooth decay to diabetes and asthma. It's called oil pulling, and it has experienced a resurgence in popularity in the past few years, probably because coconut oil (which is the typical oil of choice) is now being hailed as an all-around health promoter and more people have embraced DIY health practices (as evidenced by the 165,000 people who signed up for my Essential Oils Revolution telesummits!).

Oil pulling works by detoxifying your mouth in much the same way that soap cleans dirty dishes. Because most toxins are fat-soluble, it literally sucks contaminants—such as bacteria and small bits of food—out of your mouth and creates an antiseptic oral environment that contributes to the proper flow of saliva, which is needed to prevent cavities and disease.

OIL PULLING WITH ESSENTIAL OILS

Makes 1 application

1 drop of clove, lemon, or orange essential oil
1 tablespoon organic, unrefined coconut oil (melted), olive oil, or untoasted sesame oil

1. Add the drop of essential oil to the coconut or other oil, then pour the oil into your mouth.
2. Start lightly swishing the oil around in your mouth—do not swallow!
3. Keep going for 20 minutes. I know that may sound like a long time, but you won't even notice 20 minutes have gone by if you do this during your normal morning routine (i.e., while you shower, put on your clothes, and prep for the day).

4. Be sure *not* to spit out the mixture into your sink, or the coconut oil may end up clogging your pipes (olive oil, which gets washed down people's kitchen sinks every day, goes down fine if you run a little warm water behind it; coconut oil, on the other hand, solidifies at room temperature)—either spit it out in the trash or into a jar or some other container you can dispose of later.

5. Immediately afterward, rinse your mouth out with warm water. Don't be shocked if the oil/saliva mixture you spit out is milky white or yellow.

6. Finally, brush your teeth as normal.

Note: *This should be a relatively relaxing process, so don't think that you need to swish the oil around your mouth for the entire time—you'd wear out your jaw muscles! Simply move the oil in your mouth and through your teeth without swallowing any of it. I recommend oil pulling no more than three or four times per week.*

Also, if you're battling an infection, you may want to use 1 drop of the Immunity-Boosting Blend on page 50 instead.

3

Stocking Your Medicine Cabinet

While Jesus was having dinner at Matthew's house, many tax collectors and sinners came and ate with him and his disciples. When the Pharisees saw this, they asked his disciples, "Why does your teacher eat with tax collectors and sinners?" On hearing this, Jesus said, "It is not the healthy who need a doctor, but the sick."

—MATTHEW 9:10-11

This quote shows us that in its infancy, the medical profession was designed to serve the sick, not the healthy. The responsibility to *stay* healthy resided with each person; doctors were only consulted on how to *restore* health.

Somehow, somewhere down the line this fundamental truth shifted. Today, the medical community is seen as the primary means for not only treating disease, but preventing it.

MEDICINE IS NOT PREVENTION

I have a problem with this premise for a number of reasons. At the top of the list is the fact that medical doctors aren't trained in prevention. What they *are* highly skilled in is diagnosing and treating disease through pharmaceutical and surgical procedures.

Consider, for instance, that doctors aren't properly educated in nutrition—the foundation of health for every living being on this planet. How can someone properly help you prevent a disease if they aren't equipped with the tools necessary to help your body ward off illness and heal itself?

A 2015 survey assessed the state of nutrition education at American medical schools and compared it with recommended instructional targets.[1] Polling each of the 133 U.S. medical schools that have a four-year curriculum about the extent and type of nutrition education students are required to complete, the survey found that 71 percent of the schools fail to provide the recommended minimum 25 hours of nutrition education, and nutrition practice accounts for an average of only 4.7 hours. Moreover, what's really scary is that these numbers are trending in the wrong direction! Both the average hours of required nutrition education and the number of schools that require a nutrition course had decreased since 2000.

The researchers concluded that "U.S. medical schools still fail to prepare future physicians for everyday nutrition challenges in clinical practice. It cannot be a realistic expectation for physicians to effectively address obesity, diabetes, metabolic syndrome, hospital malnutrition, and many other conditions as long as they are not taught during medical school and residency training how to recognize and treat the nutritional root causes."[2]

That's why conventional medicine will always fail to truly help you ward off disease. Unless, of course, your health care provider has received advanced training in core concepts such as nutrition, exercise, and natural therapies like essential oils.

And you know what? This is all fine! That's not what medical doctors are there for. They are there, thank God, to help us through emergency situations and those times when natural therapies and self-help are insufficient.

The key is to keep things in proper perspective; if you want to stay well and address the root cause of disease, you've got to keep your medicine cabinet stocked with natural solutions, because you're not likely to get much help from your medical provider on these two fronts.

Here are the top essential oils to keep in your medicine cabinet to help you stay healthy.

TOP EIGHT ESSENTIAL OILS TO GET YOU STARTED

There are nearly as many essential oils as there are plants. How then, do you decide which ones to buy, especially when you're starting out? To help you avoid overbuying or stressing out in the essential oil aisle, I have listed eight of the most commonly used essential oils with the widest range of applications. Not only are these easy to find, they are also very cost-effective. Most companies offer starter kits that include all or many of these, so enjoying their therapeutic benefits should be a cinch!

Are there other essential oils that deserve a place of honor in your medicine cabinet? Absolutely—I'll cover more of them in chapter 6. But these are where you want to start. With these on hand, you will be able to make more powerful blends than you will likely ever need.

1. Lavender (*Lavandula angustifolia*)

For over 2,500 years, the medicinal and religious uses of lavender have been documented, from ancient texts through modern times. The earliest records show it was used as part of the mummification process in Egypt. Then lavender became a staple in Roman bathhouses, fragrance, and cooking. That lavender has stood the test of time, inspiring interest in so many eras, cultures, and generations, is a testament to its wide array of capabilities.

Well known for its soothing and calming properties, lavender is wonderful for accelerating the healing time for burns, cuts, stings, and other wounds. It is jam-packed with antioxidant power, and has been shown to help with sleep, anxiety, and depression. I put it first on the list because if you buy only one essential oil, lavender is the one to choose.

Here are the top five healing benefits of lavender:

1. **Potent antioxidant capabilities.** Antioxidants are just the super healers that our culture needs. The free radicals created by toxins, pollutants, chemicals, and even stress are the culprits behind a cascade of cellular damage, immune inhibition, and limitless health risks—including chronic illness and cancer. In 2012, Chinese researchers observed that lavender essential oil would upregulate all three major antioxidant enzyme levels in mice within the first day of treatment.[3] In Romania, researchers noted similar activity using inhaled lavender for an hour each day among rats.[4]

2. **Metabolism management.** In 2014, in a fifteen-day study of diabetic rats, a

lavender essential oil treatment protected against all of the following hallmarks of diabetic illness: high levels of blood glucose, metabolic illness, weight gain, depletion of antioxidants, and liver and kidney dysfunction.[5]

3. **Neurological health protection.** Lavender essential oil has long been used to beat stress, depression, and anxiety, which all fall under the umbrella of neurological conditions. Lavender's neuroprotective abilities have been confirmed time and time again, most notably in a full literature review in the *International Journal of Psychiatry in Clinical Practice* in 2013. A lavender oil preparation in gelatin capsules was shown to consistently relieve symptoms such as sleep disturbance, anxiety, and low quality of life.[6] What's more, no one reported side effects, interactions, or withdrawal symptoms. If you've ever taken pharmaceuticals for these conditions, you know how incredible that statement is!

4. **Antimicrobial agent.** Nearly one hundred published studies have documented lavender's role as an antimicrobial protectant against infections. Scientists from the University of the Witwatersrand, South Africa, tested forty-five blends for antimicrobial protection and discovered that synergistic blends produced the greatest result. Lavender–cinnamon leaf and lavender-orange blends were the most powerful.[7]

5. **Skin soother.** Particularly when mixed with a soothing carrier oil like aloe or coconut—at a ratio of 12 drops per 1 ounce of carrier oil—lavender essential oil is highly effective in treating sunburns, dry skin, minor scrapes and cuts, and canker sores. Even some immediate hypersensitivity allergic reactions may be mitigated with lavender![8]

Tisserand and Young's Lavender Safety Summary

- Hazards: None known
- Contraindications: None known[9]

Note: Robert Tisserand and Rodney Young's book *Essential Oil Safety: A Guide for Health Care Professionals* is the go-to resource for safety recommendations, contraindications, and dosing within the aromatherapy community. It's a vital resource for any serious aromatherapy student, and I include their safety summaries to help ensure you're aware of any potential risks associated with the oils discussed in this chapter.

Dr. Z's Safety Note: Lavender is considered one of the safest essential oils to use on the entire family. As with all oils, stick to recommended dilutions, keep clear of the eyes and the inside of the nose, and always listen to your body.

You may see reports on the Internet about how boys should avoid lavender because it can cause prepubertal gynecomastia (when boys experience enlarged, tender breast buds) for a short period of time (one to five months). The only reason you're even seeing this is because of a poorly researched 2007 *New England Journal of Medicine* article titled "Prepubertal Gynecomastia Linked to Lavender and Tea Tree Oils." It was determined that all three boys who developed breasts were using either a shampoo, lotion, soap, or balm that included lavender oil and tea tree oil as ingredients. The researchers extrapolated that these essential oils were "estrogenic" based on a preliminary in vitro evaluation.[10]

There are several epidemiological reasons why this conclusion is false and it is beyond the scope of this book to cover each one, but I'll leave you with this thought: Just because lavender and tea tree oils were two common ingredients in the products that these three boys used does not prove that they were the cause. This is an example of the classic statistics blunder that confuses correlation and causation. There were countless other variables that weren't considered—including the boys' diets, environmental triggers, and prescription medications.

Essential oils safety expert Robert Tisserand emphatically states, "Lavender oil does not mimic estrogen nor does it enhance the body's own estrogens. It is therefore not a hormone disruptor, cannot cause breast growth in young boys (or girls of any age), and is safe to use by anyone at risk for estrogen-dependent cancer."[11] This means that lavender isn't estrogenic and won't cause or complicate breast cancer. Tisserand's conclusion has been supported by more recent research.[12] The same is true for tea tree.

2. Peppermint (*Mentha piperita*)

Aside from lavender, peppermint may be the most versatile of all essential oils. It has the ability to:

- Treat a variety of illnesses, including stress, migraines, skin conditions, and digestive wellness
- Combat side effects associated with common cancer treatments
- Affect the body via respiratory, digestive, or topical applications
- Remain affordable thanks to easy propagation
- Stand up to thorough research
- Act as a soothing digestive aid, helping to prevent nausea, vomiting, and any other harsh gastrointestinal contractions during times of illness
- Provide a potential solution to antibiotic-resistant infections[13]

Here are my favorite uses for peppermint essential oil:

1. **Stop fevers.** Mama Z and I have found that nothing works to cool a fever like a blend of peppermint and orange oils. Preblend a 1:1 ratio of these two oils and mix with a carrier to 2%–3%, then apply on the back along the spine from the base of the neck to the sacrum.
2. **Ease muscle tension.** Peppermint essential oil is one of the best natural muscle relaxers and pain relievers. Try using a 2%–3% dilution on an aching back, toothache, or tension headache.
3. **Clear sinuses.** Diffusing a few drops of peppermint essential oil usually clears stubborn sinuses and soothes sore throats immediately. Used as an expectorant, the results can be long-lasting and beneficial when you're plagued with a cold, a cough, or bronchitis, asthma, or sinusitis.
4. **Relieve joint pain.** Peppermint oil and lavender oil work well together as a cooling, soothing anti-inflammatory for painful joints.
5. **Cut cravings.** Slow an out-of-control appetite by diffusing peppermint before meals, helping you feel full faster. Alternatively, rub a peppermint massage oil on your chest or back of neck between meals to keep hunger at bay.

6. **Energize naturally.** On a road trip or during a late-night study session, or anytime you get that low-energy slump, inhaling peppermint oil is a refreshing, nontoxic pick-me-up to help you wake up and keep going.

7. **Freshen shampoo.** A few drops included in your shampoo and conditioner will tingle your scalp and wake your senses. As a bonus, peppermint's antiseptic properties can also help prevent or remove both lice and dandruff.

8. **Ease allergies.** Peppermint can help relieve symptoms during allergy season by relaxing the nasal passages and acting as an expectorant. Apply a 2%–3% solution topically on the back of your neck or chest.

9. **Relieve ADHD.** A spritz of peppermint on clothing or added to your diffuser can help to improve concentration and alertness when focus is needed.

10. **Soothe an itch.** Cooling peppermint and calming lavender combine again to ease bug bites, sunburns, and even hemorrhoids. Just be sure to dilute! As a reminder, a 2% dilution is the standard, safe formulation for adults. However, I have found that using upwards of 10% can help for those really itchy spots!

11. **Block mosquitoes.** Peppermint oil has been found to repel mosquitoes that harbor malaria and filarial and yellow fever for up to three hours after application![14]

Tisserand and Young's Peppermint Safety Summary

- Hazards: Choleretic (stimulates bile production), mucous membrane irritation, and neurotoxicity risk (low)
- Contraindications: Cardiac fibrillation and G6PD deficiency. Do not apply near the face of infants.
- Cautions: Acid reflux (GERD)
- Maximum adult daily oral dose: 152 mg (about 5 drops)
- Maximum dermal use: 5.4%[15]

Dr. Z's Safety Note: You'll find many online resources saying that children shouldn't come into contact with peppermint because of potential breathing problems. Tisserand says that peppermint is best avoided altogether with children under three. For children aged three to six, diffusion and 0.5% topical applications are safe.[16] In my opinion, based on the lack of clinical research and on my personal experience raising four children and helping thousands of people across the globe use essential oils to reach their family's health goals, these recommendations are a little extreme—if you're diffusing a blend that includes peppermint in a well-ventilated room, your children should be just fine. Just don't put the diffuser next to the crib and discontinue use immediately if you notice any adverse reactions.

Regarding topical applications for kids, Mama Z and I have used highly diluted (1% or less) peppermint on our children as young as one year old for fevers. Of course, discretion is advised and, if you have any concerns, don't use it. Always have safety in mind when using oils with your children, and discontinue use and contact your pediatrician immediately if any adverse reactions occur.

3. Eucalyptus (*Eucalyptus globulus* **and** *radiata*)

Used copiously by Australian Aborigines for most maladies in their villages, eucalyptus is a potent antibacterial, antispasmodic, and antiviral agent. Like clove essential oil, eucalyptus has a profound effect on staph infections. Quite amazingly, recent research from VIT University in India showed (real-time) that when *Staphylococcus aureus* came into contact with eucalyptus oil, the deadly bacteria completely lost viability within just fifteen minutes of interaction![17]

Two of the most common varieties that you'll find on the market are *Eucalyptus globulus* and *Eucalyptus radiata*. The difference comes down to a slight distinction between therapeutic benefits and aroma, with *E. globulus* being the stronger of the two on both accounts. Still, *E. radiata* is exceptionally healing, and many users new to essential oils prefer it because of its softer and sweeter smell.

Here are seven amazing uses for eucalyptus oil:

1. **Expectorant and purifier.** When you've got a cold or the flu, you might feel like your head will explode if you can't expel mucus. Eucalyptus works as an expectorant to ease that discomfort, and as a bonus, it can help the body to remove toxins and germs that make you feel worse. Try putting a few drops

of eucalyptus essential oil into a diffuser while you sleep to help clear your breathing so you can rest. Or, for a more powerful application, put five drops into a bowl filled with hot water, then lean over it with a towel "tented" around your head. Breathe deeply for a few minutes and enjoy the relief.

2. **Scalp tonic.** Cleanse and refresh your scalp and hair with a few drops of eucalyptus mixed into coconut or olive oil. The carriers will moisturize while the eucalyptus relieves itchy skin and dandruff.

3. **Hand and foot cleanser.** Grease can't stand a chance against eucalyptus, making a strong case for its inclusion in homemade cleansers—or, if you're up for a real treat, a refreshing salt soak for hands or feet. (Refer to page 144 for the recipe for Healthy Bacteria Liquid Hand Soap.)

4. **Potent cleaning agent.** If you enjoy the fragrance of eucalyptus, you may already be including it in your cleaning recipes. It is also highly antimicrobial, helping to clear surfaces of potential germs. If you're making a cleaner of any sort, you need to add eucalyptus. (See page 160 for a recipe for Tea Tree Citrus Bathroom Cleaner, which calls for lemon eucalyptus, although you can swap it for regular ecualytpus.)

5. **Stain removal.** If you have stained fabric surfaces, give eucalyptus essential oil a try. Apply a few drops on a clean white washcloth and rub out the stain. First make sure (in an inconspicuous spot) that it's compatible with your fabric, just in case it reacts poorly to the eucalyptus oil.

6. **Air freshener.** Refresh the mind and lift the spirits by making a quick spritzer: Combine 10 drops eucalyptus oil, 10 drops witch hazel, and 10 drops organic grain alcohol (190 proof) in a 1-ounce spritzer bottle, then fill with distilled water. (Even after a long day at work this one is easy.) Simply spray throughout room and enjoy!

7. **Odor control.** After a long day of summer play, the laundry room can become quite noxious. After washing stinky clothes, throw them in the dryer with a wet rag that you've sprinkled with a few drops of eucalyptus essential oil. To remove odors from shoes, stick a rag with a few drops of eucalyptus into each shoe before setting them in a sunny spot to dry out. This helps prevent odors and keep the shape of the shoe intact!

Tisserand and Young's Eucalyptus Safety Summary

- Hazards: Essential oils rich in 1,8-cineole can cause central nervous system and breathing problems in young children.
- Contraindications: Do not apply near the face of infants or children under ten.
- Maximum adult daily oral dose: 600 mg (about 20 drops)
- Maximum dermal use: 20%[18]

Dr. Z's Safety Note: You'll find many online resources saying that children shouldn't come into contact with eucalyptus. Tisserand says that eucalyptus can be diffused or applied topically up to 0.5% on children under three years old. For children aged three to six, eucalyptus is safe to diffuse and apply topically up to 1.0%.[19] The key here is to avoid the face, as his safety summary indicates. I have listed how to calculate dilutions in chapter 2 (page 53). As with peppermint essential oils, Mama Z and I have used eucalyptus with our children within these parameters without any problem. As always, discontinue use and contact your pediatrician immediately if any adverse reactions occur.

4. Lemon (*Citrus limon*)

Various citrus essential oils are widely used to stimulate lymph drainage; rejuvenate sluggish, dull skin; and repel bugs. Lemon oil stands out, however, as research has recently discovered that it carries useful antimicrobial and anti-inflammatory properties,[20] and is even being praised for its ability to combat foodborne pathogens.[21] Lemon oil's cancer-fighting antioxidant power is impressive.

Nearly seven hundred studies have examined lemon essential oil, exploring dozens of traditional uses. Its most prominent component, d-limonene, is likely the key to its potency. Lemon essential oil also has an incredible uplifting scent that makes it an ideal addition to any cleaning-product preparations. Here are six ways to use it in your cleaning supplies:

1. **Disinfectant.** Bleach is harsh, especially when little hands and lungs are around. Instead, add 20 drops lemon oil to a mixture of 8 ounces distilled water, 8 ounces white vinegar, and 2 ounces organic grain alcohol (190 proof). Use it to clean moldy showers and germy countertops.
2. **Laundry freshener.** We've all forgotten to switch wet laundry to the dryer at least once. Just add a few drops of lemon oil in a rinse to remove that awful odor.
3. **Goo-be-gone.** Sticker books are a parent's nemesis when the stickers find a home on windows and furniture. Remove stickers, gum, and other gooey remnants with the help of lemon essential oil!
4. **Greasy hands solution.** Soap doesn't always cut it, particularly after you've been working on your car or bike. But with a couple drops of lemon essential oil added to your soap, the grime washes right off!
5. **Leather treatment.** A dab of lemon oil on a cloth will restore leather furniture, shoes, and clothing to their original shine.
6. **Silver polish.** Use the same treatment on tarnished silverware and jewelry to bring back the shine.

Tisserand and Young's Lemon (Expressed) Safety Summary

- Hazards: Risk (low) of skin sensitization if oxidized
- Contraindications (dermal): Potentially phototoxic; do not expose skin to sun or sunbed for twelve hours after topical application.
- Cautions: Avoid old, oxidized oils.
- Maximal dermal use: 2%[22]

Dr. Z's Safety Note: Take care to properly dilute lemon when consuming it in your water or using a solubilizer. When I was an essential oil newbie, I dropped lemon essential oil directly into my water and developed acid reflux. Once I discontinued use temporarily, I was fine and my heartburn quickly went away.

5. Frankincense (*Boswellia carterii, frereana, sacra,* and *serrata*)

Even though the chemistry differs among the four primary species of frankincense that you'll find on the market (*Boswellia carterii, frereana, sacra,* and *serrata*), many aromatherapists agree that their therapeutic effect is largely the same. For the most part, unless there is conclusive research to suggest otherwise, the species that you include in your favorite DIY recipes is up to preference. Personally, I like to use a blend of all four.

Known as the king of essential oils, frankincense is finally getting the attention it deserves as one of the most viable healing agents on the planet. It is a powerful anti-inflammatory agent, painkiller,[23] and immune booster,[24] and has been shown to kill cancer cells in vitro (which is a fancy way of saying "cells in a petri dish" and not in a living person or animal).

The journal *Oncology Letters* published an article in 2014 that highlights the ability of this biblical tree to kill cancer cells, specifically the MCF-7 and HS-1 cell lines, which cause breast and other tumors.[25] Studies continue to emerge, demonstrating similar effects on bladder[26] and skin[27] cancers.

Before you start picking up frankincense by the kilo, keep in mind that this study, like most of the others out there discussing how essential oils can kill cancer, is in vitro. Promising as they may be, let's put first things first and recognize that these cells-in-a-petri-dish evaluations can prove only so much. That said, I personally know numerous people who have used essential oils, including frankincense, to treat cancer with great results.

Frankincense essential oil has also been used with much success to treat issues related to digestion, the immune system, oral health, respiratory concerns, and stress/anxiety.

Tisserand and Young's Frankincense Safety Summary

- Hazards: Skin sensitization if oxidized
- Cautions: Avoid old, oxidized oils.[28]

Dr. Z's Safety Note: Don't fall into the trap of dousing yourself with frankincense and putting several drops in your mouth to prevent or kill cancer. I see way too much of this online. Yes, it's safe to use with minimal restrictions, but it's still a highly concentrated plant compound. Using common sense and following the safety recommendations outlined in chapter 2 will serve you well.

6. Rosemary (*Rosmarinus officinalis*)

Used for centuries to improve everything from memory and brain function to common aches and pains, rosemary even has a history of stimulating hair growth. But one amazing healing effect that many people are unaware of is its ability to normalize blood pressure.

In one of the few human studies evaluating this phenomenon, researchers from the Universidad Complutense de Madrid took thirty-two hypotensive patients and measured how their dangerously low blood pressure fared under rosemary essential oil treatments for seventy-two weeks. In addition to observing that rosemary could raise blood pressure to normal levels in a majority of the volunteers, the researchers discovered that overall mental and physical quality of life was drastically improved, which highlights the far-reaching healing effects that this ancient oil has on health and wellness.[29]

Another important fact about rosemary is that it can possibly attenuate cancer growth. Although we only have in vitro studies (again, studies conducted on living cells in a petri dish), researchers suggest that rosemary essential oil can help prevent and treat a variety of cancer cell lines. Of the thirty compounds in the essential oil, there are a few main players: α-pinene, borneol, (–) camphene, camphor, verbenone, and bornyl-acetate.

The study suggesting this was published in the journal *Molecules* after evaluating in vitro antibacterial activities and toxicology properties of *R. officinalis* essential oil compared to α-pinene, β-pinene, and 1,8-cineole. According to the study, "*R. officinalis* essential oil exhibited the strongest toxicity towards three different types of human cancer cells."[30]

Tisserand and Young's Rosemary Safety Summary

- Hazards: Neurotoxicity (depending on camphor levels)
- Contraindications: For the 1,8-cineole chemotype—essential oils rich in 1,8-cineole can cause central nervous system and breathing problems if applied on or near the face. Do not apply near the face of infants or children under ten.
- Maximal adult daily oral dose: Camphor ct. (513 mg), α-pinene ct. (676 mg), and verbenone ct. (192 mg)
- Maximal dermal use: Camphor ct. (16.5%), α-pinene ct. (22%), and verbenone ct. (6.5%)[31]

Dr. Z's Safety Note: Rosemary is similar to eucalyptus because of the 1,8-cineole content. You'll find some online resources saying that children shouldn't come into contact with rosemary. The key here is to avoid the face, as the safety summary just above indicates. I have listed how to calculate dilutions in chapter 2 (page 53). As with peppermint and eucalyptus essential oils, Mama Z and I have safely used rosemary with our children within these parameters. However, discontinue use and contact your pediatrician immediately if any adverse reactions occur.

7. Tea Tree (*Melaleuca alternifolia*)

Tea tree is a wound healer with a rich history of use as a local antiseptic for burns and cuts as well as treatment for a wide spectrum of bacterial and fungal infections (including athlete's foot and jock itch). Other conditions that respond well to tea tree include:

- Acne
- Chicken pox
- Cold sores
- Congestion and respiratory tract infections
- Earaches
- Fungal infections
- Halitosis
- Head lice
- Psoriasis
- Dry cuticles
- Insect bites, sores, and sunburns
- Boils from staph infections

I cover how to use tea tree to treat fungal infections in detail in chapter 15 when I discuss candida overgrowth.

Tisserand and Young's Tea Tree Safety Summary

- Hazards: Skin sensitization risk (low)
- Cautions (dermal): Avoid old, oxidized oils.
- Maximal dermal use: 15%[32]

Dr. Z's Safety Note: Because of its antimicrobial properties, people use tea tree frequently for a variety of infections. I know a man who, not knowing any better, literally put a drop of tea tree in his eye after coming down with conjunctivitis. I'm not kidding! He went to Dr. Google and found out that tea tree could help. Not reading far enough to learn that the proper application is to dab diluted tea tree *around* the socket, he put a drop directly onto his eyeball. Thankfully, he had the sense to wash his eye with coconut oil when the burning ensued.

Please be safe. Not to sound like a broken record, but using common sense and following the safety recommendations in chapter 2 will serve you well.

8. Ylang Ylang (*Cananga odorata*)

If frankincense is the king of essential oils, ylang ylang is the queen. From diabetes to hypertension to anxiety to (fill in the blank), ylang ylang can cover it all! It is exceptionally adept at combating depression, free radicals, inflammation, bacteria and fungi, insects, and excess melanin, which can cause skin disorders (antimelanogenesis).[33]

Interestingly, ylang ylang has the uncanny ability to be a harmonizer. According to one study that tested how twenty-four healthy adults responded to ylang ylang aromatherapy, it caused a significant decrease in blood pressure and pulse rate as well as a significant increase in attentiveness and alertness.[34] This is profound because, by definition, pulse rate and blood pressure increase when someone's fight-or-flight response kicks in, causing them to become alert and ultra-attentive. In this case, however, ylang ylang increased attentiveness and alertness without the fight-or-flight trigger, debunking the myth that it's a "calming" oil. It is a whatever-you-need kind of oil and can help the body meet the need(s) that it's facing!

Ylang ylang is the perfect example of how essential oils can balance conflicting physiological actions and truly "harmonize" the body.

Tisserand and Young's Ylang Ylang Safety Summary

- Hazards: Skin sensitization risk (moderate)
- Contraindications (dermal): Damaged, diseased, or hypersensitive skin and children under two years
- Maximal dermal use: 0.8%[35]

Dr. Z's Safety Note: Consuming high doses of ethanolic extracted ylang ylang root bark has been shown to have spermatotoxic effects.[36] As a result, researchers are investigating whether it can be a viable natural contraceptive. The particular study in question tested 1 gram of ylang ylang per kilogram of body weight per day on male rats for sixty days, which is about 2.5 ounces. The likelihood of your consuming this much or even applying the topical equivalent is slim to none. However, as ylang ylang is a common oil in women's blends and libido-boosting solutions, if you're trying to have a baby, you probably don't want to use a massage oil containing ylang ylang oil as a lubricant.

So, what do you think? Feel empowered to start tackling these eight highly versatile, power-packed essential oils? Knowing which oils to use for specific health conditions takes practice, but trust me: It'll be worth it!

4

Quick-Start Guide to Using Essential Oils to Change Your Life

The greatest medicine of all is to teach people not to need it.

—*HIPPOCRATES*

During the first essential oils class that I taught, a woman in the audience interrupted me when I started to cover certain blends and oils known to help with mood disorders. I could see her in the back of the small audience, eyes all lit up with excitement as she blurted out, "Those oils helped me get off my anxiety meds five years ago!"

She went on to talk about how nothing else had worked and how she had been beside herself, not knowing what to do. Still, she took the drugs her doctor prescribed because she felt they were her only hope. And then she met essential oils. It was wonderful to hear her tell us that essential oils helped her to live again.

What impressed me most was not that she found a natural solution to her problem, but that as a regular oil user for more than five years, she was still going to beginning 101 classes to learn all she could about how to use essential oils to enhance her life. She was a living example that there is always more to learn, and that no matter how much you think you know, you can always be a student and deepen your understanding.

HOW HUNGRY ARE YOU FOR CHANGE?

I hope you come to realize (if you haven't already) that you aren't at the mercy of your doctor, pharmacist, liquor store owner, or cigarette manufacturer. You have control over your own health and, best of all, taking control doesn't have to be hard work.

I'm guessing you've probably heard that essential oils are great for making your own nontoxic cleaning products and all-natural alternatives to air fresheners. While these *are* common and beneficial uses for essential oils—who wouldn't want to reduce their exposure to toxic chemicals and save money while doing it?—most people aren't aware of how much power essential oils have to improve their health and well-being.

Essential oils are incredible healers. Some people, including that woman I met at my first class, consider them superheroes—picture a little dark bottle with a cape flying in the air on its way to save a city under attack by aliens. OK, that may be a bit of a stretch, but that's how the millions of folks who have been able to come off their anxiety meds, blood pressure pills, and harsh anti-inflammatories regard essential oils.

Essential oils can help you sleep better, relieve your pain, heal your digestion, support you in losing weight, and help you feel vibrant enough to pursue abundant and radiant health in all areas of your life. Maybe that superhero image isn't too much of an exaggeration after all?

The blessing and the curse of essential oils is that there are innumerable applications of these little superheroes and you could spend a lifetime learning all of the ins and outs. The depth of information and range of possibilities can be overwhelming, so I want to give you some quick and easy-to-understand instruction targeted at creating big changes in your health.

While I hope you'll become a lifelong student of essential oils, I also know that your commitment will grow if you experience some of their transformative powers in your own life. To that end, I want to share with you the seven steps that I have found to be the most effective ways to start experiencing their many benefits right away. Start by choosing just one of these areas to focus on, then move on to the next once you've noticed a positive shift. After you make improvements in these foundational areas, you can go on to troubleshoot your specific symptoms and conditions with the information provided in the later chapters of this book.

I think you'll be delighted at how just a few oils and techniques can have such a noticeable impact on your overall well-being, and I trust that you'll want to keep deepening your experience of the power of essential oils to heal.

STEP 1: GET A BETTER NIGHT'S SLEEP

Getting a better night's sleep is arguably the most overlooked but effective way to keep your body healthy. Without it, you'll never be able to recuperate and regenerate from a long day full of stressors and worries.

Using essential oils to help you get the sleep your body needs can be as easy as rubbing some diluted lavender oil on your skin. Research has shown that topical application of lavender mixed with a carrier oil may actually be one of the most effective methods for people with sleep disorders, as the chemical components of lavender have been shown to enter the bloodstream within five minutes of massaging the oil on the skin.[1] And if you are worried about lavender being a long-lasting sedative that will make you groggy upon waking, know that the same study showed that most of the lavender was eliminated from the bloodstream within ninety minutes.

As I've seen with several people I've worked with, lavender oil can potentially help you get off those dangerous over-the-counter and prescription sleep remedies. Based on a clinical study dating back to 1995, we have known that sleep duration significantly decreases in elderly patients who are dependent on benzodiazepines. However, once lavender essential oil aromatherapy was introduced into their lives, their sleep quality and duration were restored to previous levels, in spite of not being on the drugs. Best of all, unlike common sleep aids and benzodiazepines, there are virtually no side effects when people use lavender or other calming essential oils to help with sleep when they use it the right way.[2]

Try this: Mix 1 drop lavender oil with 1 teaspoon fractionated coconut oil and massage over your abdomen (because it's one of the most absorbent parts of your body) before going to sleep tonight.

STEP 2: REDUCE STRESS

Without peace, there is chaos. Stress is not only the prime instigator of chaos, but is arguably the primary cause of most chronic disease today and is public enemy number one in my book. As a recent study out of Taiwan suggests, workplace stress-related illness is reaching epidemic proportions, and the ability of essential oils to directly affect the stress response by reducing blood pressure, lessening heart rate variability, and balancing other autonomic nervous system measures is profound.[3] (The autonomic nervous system is responsible for controlling vital functions not consciously directed, such as breathing, heartbeat, and digestion.)

Lavender is the trusty stalwart of stress relief, but it's not the only game in town. Just a small amount of sandalwood essential oil can help to calm anxious, restless nerves in any situation. Because sources of stress vary, you also want a variety of stress reducers so you can find the one that works best for you. Geranium, neroli, ylang ylang, and spikenard all have impressive research results that attest to their abilities to calm and soothe.

Try this: Next time you feel stressed out, simply open up a bottle of ylang ylang, spikenard, or neroli and take a few deep breaths through your nose with your eyes closed while meditating on something positive.

STEP 3: BOOST MOOD

Your sense of smell, which is part of the olfactory system, is the only sense that is controlled by the amygdala and the limbic system—the parts of your brain that play a role in mood and emotions.[4] The direct connection between scent and the limbic system is likely why scent triggers memory, as well as why certain scents have such powerful effects on mood. Of particular note when it comes to improving mood are rose and peppermint essential oils. Rose and citrus oils such as lemon appear time and again in studies demonstrating the ability of essential oils to uplift mood, trigger relaxation, and relieve anxiety.[5] And minty fresh peppermint oil also buoys your brain when you're feeling down, big-time. As an added bonus, peppermint essential oil is a natural headache treatment—and who can be in a good mood when your head hurts?

Try this: Next time you're down in the dumps, put 2 drops each of lemon, lime, and bergamot essential oils in your diffuser and enjoy a nice boost in your mood.

STEP 4: CLEAR BRAIN FOG

Like it or not, people of all ages—from kids to postmenopausal women—are experiencing less-than-clear thinking, ranging from general brain fog to ADHD (attention deficit hyperactivity disorder). Essential oils can be effective for relieving symptoms of ADHD and helping kids (or adults!) to focus. Vetiver,[6] peppermint, and rosemary are particularly effective. Rosemary has been known as the "herb of remembrance" for centuries and has been shown to improve memory and recall in adults and to improve orientation in older patients suffering with dementia.[7]

Try this: Make my Focus and Clarity Inhaler for on-the-go mental alertness when you need it most!

FOCUS AND CLARITY INHALER
10 drops rosemary essential oil
5 drops pine essential oil
5 drops *Litsea cubeba* (also known as may chang) essential oil

SUPPLIES
Precut organic cotton pad
Aromatherapy inhaler

1. Place a cotton pad in the inhaler tube.
2. Drop the essential oils directly onto the cotton pad in the tube. Alternatively, you can drop the essential oils into a glass bowl, roll the cotton pad in the oils to absorb them, and then insert it into the inhaler tube using tweezers.
3. Open the inhaler and take a few deep breaths through your nose with your

eyes closed. Repeat as often as needed whenever you need a quick boost of mental clarity.

Note: *Though they are not as common to most people's medicine cabinets and are new to our discussion, I have found that pine and Litsea cubeba (aka may chang) essential oils—traditionally known for their uplifting, grounding properties—create a nice blend with rosemary to promote focus and clarity.*

Alternatively, if you don't have these on hand, you can replace them with any oils that can help reduce clouded thinking, such as eucalyptus, peppermint, and spearmint. To find a more exhaustive list of oils to help increase alertness, check out my "Morning Ritual: Get Up and Go Practice" in chapter 5.

To watch me make this Focus and Clarity Inhaler and to learn more about beating brain fog with essential oils, go to HealingPowerOfEssentialOils.com.

STEP 5: BALANCE HORMONES

Women's hormones are true gifts from God as they make the gift of new life possible, but they are all too commonly accompanied by burdensome symptoms, including mood swings, bloating, irritation, fatigue, and depression. Although these symptoms are common, they don't have to be a given. Essential oils provide a proven alternative to the synthetic hormones so often prescribed in the form of birth control pills or hormone replacement therapy.

Young women dealing with menstrual pain have found relief by using essential oils, even beyond what acetaminophen can provide.[8] Women with dysmenorrhea have found similar relief.[9] As women reach their menopausal years, the use of antidepressants begins to increase dramatically. Clary sage may help to ease this stressful transition, reducing cortisol levels and exhibiting an antidepressant-like effect.[10]

Neroli oil, which comes from the blossoms of orange trees, has also been proven to help manage symptoms that arise from hormonal imbalance. In 2014, Korean researchers focused on neroli essential oil's impact on the symptoms of menopause, with good results. Just by inhalation, neroli was found to have a positive impact on stress relief, sexual desire, and blood pressure.[11]

Try this: Review the chapters in part 3, Women's Health, to find a natural solution for your hormone-related condition.

STEP 6: CONQUER FOOD CRAVINGS AND LOSE WEIGHT

Nothing can derail your journey toward experiencing abundant health and wellness like uncontrollable food cravings and weight gain. Thankfully, essential oils can help.

In a 2014 study published in the journal *Autonomic Neuroscience*, grapefruit and lavender oils were evaluated for their ability to affect autonomic function. Maybe you've heard of the phrases *fight or flight* and *rest and digest*. This refers to the sympathetic (which rules the fight-or-flight response) and parasympathetic (which rules the rest and digest functions of the body) nervous systems, which greatly regulate the functions of our metabolism and internal organs such as the heart, intestines, and stomach.

It was discovered that inhaling grapefruit essential oil decreases food intake and stimulates lipolysis (breakdown of fats) and thermogenesis (use of calories to produce body heat). Interestingly, lavender performs in the exact opposite way, presumably due to its relaxing, parasympathetic properties. Thus, grapefruit oil is a fantastic natural remedy to help curb unhealthy hungry cravings and help you manage your weight.[12] This study also highlights that, if someone wants to lose weight, it would be wise to avoid diffusing lavender during meals as it can increase appetite and slow down the calorie-burning process. Don't worry about using it at night, because the effects of essential oils are short-lived, up to ninety minutes, and diffusing lavender for a better night's sleep shouldn't prevent you from losing weight.

Try this: Put 1 drop of grapefruit oil and some liquid stevia extract into a 32-ounce glass bottle and fill with sparkling water. The carbonation will help you feel satiated and the grapefruit will add a nice fat-burning flavor enhancement! Be sure to avoid lavender during the daytime.

STEP 7: EASE PAIN

Let's talk about an important word in medicine today that you might have already stumbled across in your research: *inflammation.*

Inflammation has become quite the buzzword lately, hasn't it? No wonder, because it has been linked to virtually every chronic disease, including cancer, diabetes, heart disease, and even autism! According to Mark Hyman, MD, "Autoimmune conditions are connected by one central biochemical process: A runaway immune response also known as systemic inflammation that results in your body attacking its own tissues."[13]

What exactly is inflammation?

Generally speaking, inflammation is simply your immune system's natural response to a stimulus such as bacteria, viruses, cuts, scrapes, chemicals, radiation, and virtually anything that your body sees as a threat, including stress and toxic emotions.[14]

For the most part, diseases that cause inflammation end in the suffix *-itis.* Common illnesses like bronchitis (inflammation of your bronchi) and otitis media (inflammation of your middle ear) are household names at this point. These are known as *acute conditions,* which means they usually come on suddenly and are short-lived, but can persist well beyond what they should depending on how your body fights them off.

You have undoubtedly experienced acute inflammation, which is usually accompanied by one or more of these cardinal signs:

- Redness
- Heat
- Swelling
- Loss of function
- Pain

Let's focus on that last symptom. Inflammation is at the heart of most painful conditions, from injuries to chronic illness. For this reason, anti-inflammatory oils are important tools when fighting pain, whether from a headache, general muscle stiffness, or a condition such as arthritis. Thankfully, there are plenty to choose from, including copaiba, frankincense, balsam/white fir, and peppermint.

It has been suggested that essential oils with monoterpenes (a type of volatile molecule)—which, as one study notes, can comprise about 90 percent of essential oils—have some level of anti-inflammatory ability.[15] So, you have a great many options when it comes to naturally addressing pain with oils. Just be sure to always dilute the essential oil in a carrier oil as described on page 52!

Try this: Try the inflammation-soothing recipes in chapter 16. I cover this topic at great length there.

5

Getting Started: Your Essential Oils Daily Practice

A nail is driven out by another nail. Habit is overcome by habit.

—DESIDERIUS ERASMUS OF ROTTERDAM

f you came over to my house for a friendly get-together or holiday dinner you would think that Mama Z and I have it all together. Appetizers start at 4:30 p.m. and dinner begins at 5:00. By the time dinner rolls out, though, most of us are not hungry because we've already indulged in Sabrina's enticing smorgasbord of hors d'oeuvres.

It's not just the food that Sabrina spends time and energy on—it's also the ambiance. Diffusers are running all over the house to set the mood, and she always seems to find a tasteful way to display some new DIY formulation that she's working on.

We hear a lot of things from our guests like: *You mean all of THIS is healthy? You made it all from scratch?* and *I could never do that!*

And you know what? They're correct! They *can't* do what Mama Z does. At least, not if they tried without any practice. It has taken my wife more than a decade of learning from culinary failures and testing countless new recipes to get to where she is now.

I hear similar things online from folks about my lifestyle: *Dr. Z, I could never do all that your website tells me to do.*

Yes, you're right! It takes time to build healthy habits, and I've been living this way of life for more than fifteen years! It has taken me tons of trial and error, prayer, and hard work. But the good news is that at this point, it no longer feels like effort, because most of what I do, I do out of habit.

THE SCIENCE OF DEVELOPING A HEALTHY HABIT

Do you know how long it takes to create a healthy habit? It's not three weeks as you've often heard. That myth was started in the 1960s by Dr. Maxwell Maltz in his book *Psycho-Cybernetics*. With his book selling millions of copies in more than a dozen languages, it's no wonder that Maltz's theory became accepted as fact and was the mantra of countless self-help and health experts who have hit the scene in the past fifty years.

The science of forming habits actually suggests that it can take more than two months before a new, healthy behavior becomes automatic. In fact, according to a landmark study published in 2010 in the *European Journal of Social Psychology*, it takes on average sixty-six days.[1]

The study examined the behaviors of nearly a hundred people over a twelve-week period. Each person chose one new health-related habit to focus on—like drinking a bottle of water with lunch or running before dinner for fifteen minutes—and reported each day about whether they accomplished what they set out to do and whether or not the behavior felt automatic. Some people in the study reached this point in as few as eighteen days, but others took as long as 254 days, highlighting that it can take a considerable amount of time to develop a new habit, and that there is no universal standard.[2]

I like this study because it encourages us to stop comparing ourselves to others and to do the best that we can. As an online biblical health educator, I find myself filling the role of a counselor and teacher in my followers' lives. I regularly encourage people, stressing the importance of being patient with themselves and accepting temporary setbacks and failures as a necessary part of the journey.

For those of you willing to take the time to form the habit of using essential oils to enhance your life, I have developed a tried-and-true daily practice for you to follow.

CREATING NEW DAILY HABITS WITH ESSENTIAL OILS

I've devised two different ways that you can create a daily essential oils practice that suits you and your fundamental needs: a two-step morning practice to set yourself up for mental, physical, and spiritual health throughout the day; and a three-step evening practice to ensure you get a good seven hours of sleep. If you are wondering if you can commit, try it for just one day. I think you'll love it and want to do it the next day, and the next, and the next, until essential oils are part of *every* day!

For the morning practice, you have two choices:

1. If you're like Mama Z, who is an early riser by nature, and you have extra time in the morning to pray, meditate, or read God's word, then my Essential Oil Prayer and Spiritual Practice is for you. It's easy to follow using one (or all!) of the four easy-to-make recipes below.
2. If you're more like me, and you barely have enough time to shower before rushing off to get your kids to school, I'm guessing you'd rather pray or meditate later in the day. I have created a Get Up and Go Practice just for you to help make your morning transition a little more enjoyable!

Whichever kind of person you are, the blends that you create for your morning ritual can also be used at any time of the day or night when you need a quiet moment. Keep a bottle in your purse, your desk drawer, or your glove compartment so that you have it on hand.

Morning Ritual: Essential Oil Prayer and Spiritual Practice

Nothing can help you focus and get into a spiritual, meditative mindset at the beginning of the day like using essential oils. Making modern-day versions of ancient holy anointing oil recipes can help you find inner peace, calm anxiety, alleviate stress, combat depression, and balance your emotions. You can do this with either a diffuser or a roll-on applicator—I include techniques for both.

To make a morning meditation blend that will work for you, use those oils that help you reach a mindful state and combine them to create a pleasant aroma—one that you'll want to use over and over again.

Here's a list of some of the oils that have traditionally been used for mental clarity, meditation, and mindfulness. Chances are you have a couple of these on hand!

Amyris (aka West Indian
    rosewood or Indies
    sandalwood)
Angelica root
Bergamot
Buddha wood
Cedarwood
Frankincense
Elemi
Helichrysum
Key lime
Lavender
Lemon
Lime
Myrrh

Neroli
Opoponax
Orange, sweet
Palmarosa
Palo santo
Patchouli
Peru alsam
Petitgrain
Roman chamomile
Rose
Rosemary
Sandalwood
Vitex
Valerian
Ylang ylang

Try blending some of the citrus (such as lemon, lime, neroli, or orange) with the resins (frankincense, myrrh, or opoponax). Or blend some of the florals (lavender, rose, or ylang ylang) with the barks (cedarwood, sandalwood, or Peru balsam).

At first, limit your blend to two or three oils; then build your way up to six at the most.

If you need a kick start or a little more guidance, try my favorite combination: frankincense, patchouli, vetiver, ylang ylang, and neroli (or yuzu as the citrus scent). I love it!

MORNING MEDITATION DIFFUSER BLEND

**1 drop each of frankincense, patchouli, vetiver, ylang ylang, and neroli
  essential oils**

SUPPLIES
Diffuser

1. Fill the diffuser with water as directed in the instructions for your diffuser.
2. Add the essential oils.
3. Turn on the diffuser 5 minutes before you begin your prayer and spiritual practice to permeate the room with the aroma.
4. Turn off the diffuser when done.

Note: *You can keep this mixture in the diffuser and use it every morning until the diffuser is empty.*

MORNING MEDITATION INHALER

If you're on the road and don't have a diffuser on hand, then using an inhaler is the next best thing. It's also a great alternative to the diffuser if you're sensitive to smell and want to control how much of the essential oil vapors you're breathing in during your practice.

5 drops frankincense essential oil
5 drops vetiver essential oil
3 drops patchouli essential oil
3 drops ylang ylang essential oil
3 drops neroli essential oil

SUPPLIES
Precut organic cotton pad
Aromatherapy inhaler

1. Place a cotton pad in the inhaler tube.

2. Drop the essential oils directly onto the cotton pad inside the tube. Alternatively, you can drop the essential oils into a glass bowl, roll the cotton pad in the oils to absorb them, and then insert it into the inhaler tube using tweezers.

3. Open the inhaler, close your eyes, and take a few deep breaths right before you begin your meditation practice or prayer time.

MORNING MEDITATION BODY OIL

5 drops frankincense essential oil

5 drops vetiver essential oil

5 drops patchouli essential oil

5 drops ylang ylang essential oil

2 drops neroli essential oil

2 ounces carrier oil of choice or Mama Z's Oil Base (page 43)

SUPPLIES
Medium glass bowl
Lotion dispenser or glass jar

1. Drop the essential oils into a bowl.

2. Add a carrier oil and mix.

3. Use as a body oil after you shower to moisturize and help get you in the mood to pray and meditate.

4. Be sure to switch to another blend every other month.

5. Store in a lotion dispenser or glass jar.

Note: *Did you know that your body is on a monthly cycle? Your skin actually regenerates approximately every four weeks, which is one of the reasons why I am a firm believer in mixing up our protocols every month or so. The other reason is that I want to keep my body guessing—ensuring that I don't contribute to resistance. The last thing I want to do is to overdo an intervention and make my body so used to something that I need to double up the dosage to get the same effect.*

MORNING MEDITATION ROLL-ON

If a simple roll-on is more your style instead of a body oil, try this roller bottle recipe to help put you in a more prayerful, meditative mindset.

2 drops frankincense essential oil

2 drops vetiver essential oil

2 drop patchouli essential oil

2 drops ylang ylang essential oil

2 drops neroli essential oil

Enough of your favorite carrier oil to fill the glass bottle—fractionated coconut oil, jojoba, or sweet almond all work great!

SUPPLIES

10 ml glass roller bottle

1. Pour your essential oils into the bottle.
2. Fill the bottle with your favorite carrier oil.
3. Mix by shaking vigorously for 10 seconds.
4. Apply on key trigger points like wrists, behind the knees, back of the neck, and soles of the feet first thing in the morning, before your prayer time.

Morning Ritual: Get Up and Go Practice

If you're like me and you find it more enjoyable to pray and meditate later in the day, then you might enjoy a nice Get Up and Go Blend to give you energy, boost your mood, and create an uplifting aroma that you'll want to use over and over again.

Here's a list of some of the oils that have traditionally been used to increase alertness and get you ready to move.

Bay laurel	Grapefruit	Lemon tea tree
Bergamot	Key lime	Lemon myrtle
Camphor	Lemon	Lemongrass
Eucalyptus	Lemon eucalyptus	Lime

Litsea cubeba (aka may chang)	Peppermint	Rosemary
	Pine	Spearmint
Mountain savory	Ravensara	Tea tree
Orange	Ravintsara	Wintergreen

MORNING GET UP AND GO DIFFUSER BLEND

3 drops orange essential oil

2 drops peppermint essential oil

1 drop rosemary essential oil

SUPPLIES

Diffuser

1. Fill the diffuser with water as directed.

2. Add the essential oils.

3. Turn on the diffuser immediately upon rising in the morning to permeate the room with the aroma as you get ready for the day.

4. Turn off the diffuser when done. You can keep this mixture in the diffuser and use it every morning until the diffuser is empty.

➡ To watch a video demo of the Morning Get Up and Go Diffuser Blend and pick up some tips for starting your day off right, go to HealingPowerOfEssentialOils.com.

MORNING GET UP AND GO INHALER

10 drops orange essential oil

6 drops peppermint essential oil

4 drops rosemary essential oil

SUPPLIES

Precut organic cotton pad

Aromatherapy inhaler

1. Place a cotton pad in the inhaler tube.

2. Drop the essential oils directly onto the cotton pad inside the tube. Alternatively, you can drop the essential oils into a glass bowl, roll the cotton pad in the oils to absorb them, and then insert it into the inhaler tube using tweezers.

3. When you first wake up but are still in bed, open the inhaler and take a few deep breaths. Then jump right out of bed and inhale a few more times while standing up to increase blood flow and energy to your body.

MORNING GET UP AND GO BODY OIL

12 drops orange essential oil
4 drops peppermint essential oil
2 drops rosemary essential oil
2 ounces carrier oil or Mama Z's Oil Base (page 43)

SUPPLIES
Medium glass bowl
Lotion dispenser or glass jar

1. Drop the essential oils into a glass bowl.

2. Add a carrier oil and mix.

3. Use as a body oil after you shower for a cooling, power-packed energy booster.

4. Be sure to switch to another blend every other month.

5. Store in a lotion dispenser or glass jar.

MORNING GET UP AND GO ROLL-ON

Instead of using the body oil, try this roller bottle recipe to help energize and get you up and running!

5 drops orange essential oil
3 drops peppermint essential oil
1 drop rosemary essential oil

Enough of your favorite carrier oil to fill the roller bottle, such as fractionated coconut oil, jojoba, or sweet almond

SUPPLIES
10 ml glass roller bottle

1. Add the essential oils to the bottle.
2. Fill the bottle with your favorite carrier oil.
3. Mix by shaking vigorously for 10 seconds.
4. Apply on key trigger points like the wrists, behind the knees, back of the neck, and soles of the feet right after getting out of bed.

Evening: Winding Down for Rejuvenating Sleep

If you're not waking up every day refreshed and ready to tackle the day, chances are you are not getting quality sleep. Regular restorative sleep is one of the most overlooked aspects of the abundant life.

To help you set the tone for evening and prepare your body for a better night's sleep, try the following three-step nightly bedtime routine. In addition, consider keeping a gratitude journal of the things that you are thankful for as part of your nightly routine. This list will serve you well during those moments when all hell breaks loose and nothing seems to be going the right way in your life.

RESTFUL EVENING DETOX BATH

You may not have time for a full-fledged bath every night before bedtime, but taking even one detox bath each week will help your body process the stresses—and toxins!—you encounter each day. This should be the first step in your nightly bedtime ritual.

3 drops lavender essential oil
2 drops Roman chamomile oil
2 drops ylang ylang

1 tablespoon jojoba oil
1 cup Epsom salts (plain)
¼ cup organic apple cider vinegar

SUPPLIES
Medium glass bowl

1. Mix the essential oils and jojoba oil in a glass bowl.
2. Add the Epsom salts and vinegar and mix.
3. Fill your bathtub with the warmest water you can stand.
4. Slowly pour the oil/vinegar mixture into the running water.
5. Soak your whole body for 20 to 30 minutes.
6. Exit the bath slowly by first sitting up, then kneeling, and finally standing to prevent feeling faint.

RESTFUL EVENING BODY OIL

After your bath, I recommend applying some lavender or vetiver massage oils—the two most popular and effective essential oils for aiding sleep.

10 drops lavender or vetiver essential oil, or 5 drops of each
6 drops clary sage essential oil
4 drops sweet marjoram essential oil
2 ounces carrier oil or Mama Z's Oil Base (page 43)

SUPPLIES
Medium glass bowl
Lotion dispenser or glass jar

1. Drop the essential oils into a glass bowl.
2. Add a carrier oil and mix.
3. Use as a body oil after your detox bath.
4. Be sure to switch to another blend every other month.
5. Store in a lotion dispenser or glass jar.

RESTFUL EVENING ROLL-ON BLEND

As an alternative to the body oil, use this roller bottle recipe to help promote a better night's sleep.

6 drops lavender or 6 drops vetiver essential oil, or 3 drops of each
3 drops clary sage essential oil
2 drops sweet marjoram essential oil
Fractionated coconut oil or carrier oil of choice

SUPPLIES
10 ml glass roller bottle

1. Drop the essential oils into the roller bottle.
2. Fill the roller bottle with a carrier oil and shake well.
3. Massage your neck, shoulders, hands, wrists, feet, and ankles with the oil before bed.
4. While spending a few minutes giving yourself a gentle massage, reflect on the day and focus on at least one thing that you are grateful for.

RESTFUL EVENING DIFFUSER BLEND

3 drops lavender essential oil
2 drops clary sage essential oil
1 drop sweet marjoram essential oil

SUPPLIES
Diffuser

1. Fill the diffuser with water as directed.
2. Add the essential oils.
3. Turn on the diffuser 10 to 20 minutes before you go to bed.
4. Set the diffuser to run through the night.

RESTFUL EVENING INHALER

10 drops lavender essential oil

6 drops clary sage essential oil

4 drops sweet marjoram essential oil

SUPPLIES

Precut organic cotton pad

Aromatherapy inhaler

1. Place a cotton pad in the inhaler tube.
2. Drop the essential oils directly onto the cotton pad in the tube. Alternatively, you can drop the essential oils into a glass bowl, roll the cotton pad in the oils to absorb them, and then insert it into the inhaler tube using tweezers.
3. While in bed, open the inhaler and take deep breaths for about 2 minutes.

BE PATIENT WITH YOURSELF

If you struggle with creating new healthy habits, my hope and prayer is that you are patient with yourself, understanding that it takes time. Remember—no matter how many times you fall, you can always get back up again. Otherwise, you may fall into the trap of being too hard on yourself and give up trying altogether.

I'm convinced that this is one of the most common reasons why people don't use natural therapies like essential oils more often to treat their health conditions. Prescription drugs are an easy fix, whereas it may take time to master using essential oils to heal what ails you. But as with most things in life, this journey is an ongoing journey. What I present in this book is fundamentally different from conventional medicine and a whole new way of living. I hope you will embrace this approach.

6

Expanding Your Medicine Cabinet

It's hard to believe that I have gone from needing so many medications and having radiation and chemo to having just my essential oils and not needing anything else. And my oncologist is totally floored by it.

—YVONNE R.

One of Sabrina's closest friends was diagnosed with one of the deadliest forms of cancer last year. In June 2016, Yvonne felt great, living the American dream with the love of her life, raising her beautiful fifteen-year-old daughter, and running a thriving insurance business. Just a few weeks later, however, her life turned upside down. After coughing up blood during a family vacation in July, Yvonne went to the hospital, where she learned that she had stage IV non-small-cell lung cancer. Her entire life fell into a downward spiral. The cancer metastasized quickly into her brain, then throughout her spine and entire body, and she was literally on death's door by December. That's when her oncologist stopped medical treatments because her platelet levels were too low (down to 9.0) and her white blood count was at 0.5. Her medical treatments weren't working.

Her oncologist didn't want to tell her that she was dying so he broke the news to her husband, Scott, and asked him to relay the message. But Scott and Yvonne didn't give up. "This is when we took matters into our own hands," Scott told me in our interview for my podcast last year. With hope that could only be birthed in faith in the healing power of God, Scott and Yvonne prayed, asked for God's guidance, and did the only thing they knew to do.

They started applying frankincense, myrrh, and lemongrass over her body up to seven times a day. By February of 2017, Yvonne's golf-ball-sized tumor on her neck had disappeared, despite her being completely off chemotherapy for more than two months.

As I write this book, Yvonne is still using essential oils regularly. Her oncologist added immunotherapy to her regime and her total body cancer levels are decreasing. In fact, there is no cancer detectable in her brain or lungs. She's gained back most of the weight she lost. She eats a healthy diet, can walk again, has regained her eyesight, and is on the road to recovery!

Since then, Yvonne and Scott have become committed to encouraging what seems like countless friends and family members who are battling cancer. From the depths of their pain, a ministry has been born. Hallelujah!

THE IMPORTANCE OF BEING PREPARED

Ever hear of the five P's? They form a sentence: Proper planning prevents poor performance. This is the quintessence of why we all need to follow Scott's and Yvonne's instincts and make sure that we're ready for unexpected storms.

Yvonne's healing journey is a story of love, bravery, positive thinking, hope, and undying faith. It's also a story about being prepared in case things go awry.

Yvonne had a pretty solid medicine cabinet of essential oils built up by the time that she was diagnosed with cancer. I know from experience that this in and of itself is true empowerment—to be able to rest easy, knowing that you have natural solutions stockpiled just in case something goes wrong. No one likes taking middle-of-the-night trips to the twenty-four-hour pharmacy to get cough syrup, right? Same goes for essential oils!

A WORD OF CAUTION ABOUT PROTOCOLS

Think back to the days before our current paradigm, where modern technology has made the world just one click away. If you lived in Australia a thousand years ago, for example, your family lived off whatever the land provided, which meant you used tea tree and eucalyptus and other native herbs for all of your health concerns. If you lived in Haiti, you used vetiver. If you lived in France, lavender was your go-to solution. Same with Italians and citrus plants like bergamot and lemon. Our ancestors became quite adept at using what they had available within walking distance of their homes. With this in mind, remember that there is no slam-dunk essential oil that is going to work the same way for everyone. We all have a unique road to healing, and can quite possibly use different oils to achieve the same results, as our ancestors did.

Take our friends Yvonne and Scott, for example. When people hear stories like this, they have the tendency to forget about biochemical individuality and go out and buy a bunch of frankincense, lemongrass, and myrrh. Trying to follow Yvonne's unique road to healing, you could easily get discouraged and become disenchanted with essential oils if you don't experience the same results, which is completely understandable. Ignoring the possibility that your body may require something different, I'd hate for you to think that essential oils "don't work" and lose hope.

Truth be told, there are dozens of oils that have anticancer properties. So don't just go out and stock up on the same oils as Yvonne. Remember my early emphasis on biochemical individuality? There is no guarantee that the remedies I mention in this book will have the same effects on everyone. It's important to build on the information provided here by continuing to do your own research. Since essential oils research is constantly evolving, this book by no means contains everything there is to know about essential oils. Equally important is to keep trying different approaches, listening to your own body, and responding accordingly.

SELECTING THE ESSENTIAL OILS TO EXPAND YOUR MEDICINE CABINET

Once you're comfortable with a selection of basic essential oils, you'll want to keep adding to your repertoire. The list below builds on the oils that I discussed in chapter 3. These options are widely available and make it possible for you to address a broad range of needs, from cooking and cleaning to preventing illness.

If you want to make specialty blends or DIY recipes, you may need to expand beyond this list, but for the most part, these oils plus the ones in chapter 3 will get you where you want to go.

Unlike in chapter 3, where I discuss the most popular healing oils in detail, the list below is more of a quick snapshot of the oils that would help you round out your medicine cabinet to handle an even wider array of challenges. In the upcoming chapters, I'll show you how to use these fourteen oils to approach dozens of your health concerns naturally and provide more than 150 specific recipes so that you can start using them immediately. Of course, safety, dosage, and contraindication considerations still apply. For Tisserand's safety summaries for all of these oils, see *Essential Oil Safety: A Guide for Health Care Professionals, 2nd edition*.

1. **Bergamot** (*Citrus bergamia*). With more than one hundred studies investigating its effects to date, bergamot is one of the more researched oils. It has a long list of benefits, from weight loss[1] to stress relief[2] to antibacterial action.[3] Some of us like to call it "liquid Xanax" because of its widely touted—and proven—abilities to significantly lessen anxiety.[4]

2. **Clary sage** (*Salvia sclarea*). A *big* one for women's health, clary sage essential oil contains many components known for their anti-inflammatory and calming benefits, including linalool (a major component of lavender essential oil), linalyl acetate (excellent for anti-inflammatory benefits on the skin), and a component called sclareol, which has been shown in research experiments to have an impact on the way that cancer cells proliferate that could help to induce apoptosis (cancer cell death).[5] Aside from its anti-inflammatory abilities, clary sage is also known to be relaxing and to have antidepressant, antifungal, antimicrobial, and antioxidant properties.

3. **Clove** (*Syzygium aromaticum*). Superhigh on the ORAC scale, which rates the antioxidant value of foods and beverages, clove oil is commonly included in commercially available immune-boosting blends. Also great for oral health, clove has been shown to slow tooth decay and is a natural alternative to poisoning your toothpaste with fluoride.[6]

4. **Fennel** (*Foeniculum vulgare*). A potent healer of gut health, fennel is also extremely helpful for breastfeeding support and menstrual cramps. It has even been shown to help reduce infantile colic.[7]

5. **Geranium** (*Pelargonium graveolens*). Another go-to for women's health,

geranium oil boasts a long list of healing benefits that include reducing inflammation and being a potent antifungal agent.[8]

6. **Helichrysum** (*Helichrysum italicum*). This long-revered essential oil (there are records of it being used in ancient Greece) has a multitude of uses, including as an antibacterial, antifungal, anti-inflammatory, and antioxidant. It is a powerful antioxidant even at lower concentrations, but quite possibly its greatest power is its ability to heal skin and restore it to a more youthful appearance.[9] It's also known as "Immortelle" for this very reason.

7. **Lemon balm** (*Melissa officinalis*). This powerhouse oil has been shown to improve cognition and produce a palpable sense of calm and focus. It's also superpowerful for fighting cancer[10] and managing diabetes.[11] (As an added bonus, it's also great at repelling bugs.) Although it's one of the more cost-prohibitive oils, if you can afford to splurge, you won't be disappointed!

8. **Lemongrass** (*Cymbopogon flexuosus*). In my opinion, lemongrass is the most underappreciated oil: It has been shown to kill methicillin-resistant *Staphylococcus aureus* (MRSA) and other antibiotic-resistant bacteria. It also helps with high cholesterol, balances blood sugar, and calms anxiety—a true MVP.[12]

9. **Myrrh** (*Commiphora myrrha*). This superb wound healer is even more powerful than frankincense in fighting cancer.[13] It has a tendency to gum up and harden, so don't purchase more than you'll use within a few months. Studies have shown that myrrh exhibits cytotoxic, analgesic, anti-inflammatory, anticancer, antiparasitic, and hypolipidemic (lipid-lowering) activities.[14]

10. **Neroli** (*Citrus aurantium*). Another underappreciated oil, neroli is great for pain[15] and stress reduction.[16] A 2014 study also uncovered that it can be a powerful antiseizure and anticonvulsant natural agent.[17] Neroli is also a little pricey, so be sure to save your pennies, because it'll be worth it!

11. **Orange** (*Citrus sinensis*). One of the most abundant sources of the profoundly therapeutic d-limonene, orange essential oil tops my list of must-have remedies; it is by far one of the most economical, safe, and highly effective oils.

12. **Oregano** (*Origanum vulgare*). Often referred to as "nature's antibiotic," oregano is the go-to solution for all things related to infection: bacterial, fungal, and viral. As it contains potent medicinal properties, it also carries potent

safety risks. Always dilute oregano essential oil, or you could significantly irritate or even burn your skin!

13. **Sandalwood—Australian, East Indian, and Hawaiian** (*Santalum spicatum, album,* and *paniculatum*). Another more-expensive oil, sandalwood is great for anxiety, focus, and skin care, and works well in tandem with frankincense and myrrh on a wide array of issues, from building focus to battling cancer.[18] Like ylang ylang, it is a known "harmonizer."[19]

14. **Vetiver** (*Vetiveria zizanoides*). This supremely grounding oil promotes focus and has been shown in research to be helpful in ADHD management.[20] It's becoming one of the most popular oils today and has even proved to be a potent tick repellent![21]

HARNESS THE POWER OF SYNERGY

Essential oils work synergistically, in that their efficacy is amplified when they are blended together. The plant compounds interact with each other in such a way that they develop extraordinary healing power. Frankincense and myrrh are one such example. Each oil can treat a variety of diseases on its own, but they are often blended together for even greater effect to treat inflammatory conditions and to reduce swelling and pain.[22]

As you'll learn more in part 3, the Women's Health section, lavender and tea tree are another great example of the synergy of essential oils. These oils work wonderfully together to combat fungal infections.[23]

There appear to be an infinite number of potential synergies between essential oils, and researchers continue to try different combinations to find the best natural solutions to common ailments. In this book, I have reported on those studies, and many of the recipes in parts 2 and 3 come directly from this research.

MAKING YOUR OWN BLENDS

As you build your medicine cabinet, I wholeheartedly encourage you to make synergistic blends and see what works best for your body. Blending is more of an art than a science, and it takes some experimenting to find the right blends for you.

As an example, let's make an anti-anxiety blend from some of the oils we've discussed.

1. Start off with a small bottle suitable for the essential oils you're using and the delivery method you need for that particular recipe.
2. To choose which oils to include, think about the aromas that you already enjoy. Do you like the uplifting smell of citrus fruits? Then start off with lemon, neroli, or bergamot. Do you like more a grounded, woodsy smell? Then start with myrrh, frankincense, vetiver, or sandalwood. Maybe you're more into flowers. Then geranium, clary sage, lavender, or ylang ylang is your go-to. Or, do you enjoy herbs? Then try lemongrass, Melissa, or fennel.
3. Put a few drops of two or three different oils in the bottle and gently shake the bottle to mix them.
4. Once you've combined the oils, close your eyes and take in the aroma. How do you feel? What do you think? Do you like it?
5. Then, basing your formulation on your organoleptic evaluation (how your body perceives the oil through the senses of smell, sight, and intuition), add varying drops of each oil to suit your taste. In other words, if you get a headache after smelling a new blend, something isn't right. This is where the art and science of aromatherapy come into play, and it takes some tinkering to find that perfect blend for you.
6. Try putting a couple drops of this blend into a diffuser and let it permeate the room that you're in for a few minutes. If you discover that your mind and emotions start to settle down and your anxious thoughts have left you, then you've just found your blend!

ORANGE OIL: AN ESSENTIAL OIL SUPERSTAR

Few natural remedies can boost the mood and lift the spirits like orange essential oil. I'm 100 percent serious when I say it's like a liquid antidepressant! Just a little whiff straight out of the bottle and your brain goes to "happy thought" mode. It's no wonder, then, that orange oil is commonly used as a food flavoring and as an ingredient in body care products like deodorants, soaps, and lotions.

As you'll see below, studies have actually proven that simply inhaling orange oil can produce a cornucopia of emotional, psychological, and physical benefits. Just imagine what happens when you strategically apply it in healing ointments on your skin and use it in other creative ways!

When we discuss the healing benefits of orange oil, it is important to distinguish between the different types, as each oil produces different therapeutic effects and reacts to sunlight differently. The two exceptions are sweet orange and wild orange, which are the same species (*Citrus sinensis*). Some manufacturers label their *Citrus sinensis* "orange essential oil," some call it "sweet orange essential oil" and some call it "wild orange essential oil." The safety risks for all three types are thought to be the same because they are *Citrus sinensis* and this species is not known to be phototoxic. However, this is no guarantee. For the purposes of this book, I'm using "orange oil" and you may use the version of *Citrus sinensis* that is readily available to you.

- **Sweet or wild orange** (*Citrus sinensis*). Made from cold pressing the peel of oranges.
- **Neroli** (*Citrus aurantium*). Made from steam distilling bitter orange blossoms.
- **Bitter orange** (*Citrus aurantium*). Made from expressing the rind of bitter oranges.
- **Petitgrain** (*Citrus aurantium ssp. Amara*). Made from steam distilling the leaves and twigs of the bitter orange tree.
- **Mandarin or tangerine** (*Citrus reticulata*). Made from cold pressing the peel of fruit interchangeably called mandarins and tangerines, though technically speaking, tangerines are a subtype of mandarins with slight differences.
- **Bergamot** (*Citrus bergamia*). Made by cold pressing the rind of the fruit of a plant belonging to the Rutaceae family—a hybrid of bitter orange (*C. aurantium* L.) and lemon (*C. limon* L. Burm. f.) or possibly lime (*C. aurantifolia*).[24]

Five Ways to Heal with Orange Essential Oil

Primarily because of its rich d-limonene content (more on that to come), orange oil is truly one of the most versatile and cost-effective essential oils on the market. Just look at these five ways that orange oil can be used therapeutically:

1. Fight Cancer

The most prominent and noteworthy component of not only orange, but all citrus oils, is d-limonene, which has been shown to be a potent cancer-fighting agent. Although we cannot pinpoint the exact mechanism, research suggests that *d-limonene not only inhibits tumor growth, but triggers what's known as apoptosis (cancer cell suicide).*[25] Orange oil also contains polymethoxyflavones, phytochemicals that have been shown to slow the growth of and even kill human lung cancer.[26]

It's important to note that essential oil therapy for cancer patients is still untested and hotly debated because a vast majority of the research discussing the cancer-fighting benefits of essential oils is based on in vitro studies (cells in a petri dish) or conducted on animals. Granted, there are relatively few side effects if used safely and wisely—but consult your physician to make sure these oils are not contraindicated for any drugs you are taking.

Application: Prepare a citrus power-packed cancer-fighting roll-on mixed with essential oils containing carvacrol, the monoterpene that gives oregano and thyme their antimicrobial and immune-boosting properties.

CANCER-FIGHTING ROLL-ON

2 drops grapefruit essential oil
2 drops orange essential oil
2 drops tangerine essential oil
2 drops oregano essential oil
2 drops thyme essential oil
1 drop winter savory essential oil

Carrier oil of choice—jojoba and fractionated coconut oil absorb quickly and work best—as needed

SUPPLIES
10 ml glass roller bottle

1. Drop the essential oils into the roller bottle.
2. Fill the roller bottle with your carrier oil of choice and shake well.
3. Apply once or twice per day over the tumor area if isolated, or over the abdomen if the cancer is metastatic.

Note: *Do not use for prolonged periods of time; switch up every month or so as is our general rule of thumb for all protocols. You can also try other cancer-fighting oils or use different proportions to this recipe. Discontinue use immediately if redness, soreness, or pain occurs. Other well-known cancer-fighting oils include clary sage, clove, frankincense, lemongrass, Melissa, myrrh, and sandalwood.*

→ To watch me make this Cancer-Fighting Roll-On and to learn more about essential oils and cancer, go to HealingPowerOfEssentialOils.com.

2. Improve Cognitive Function

An interesting study published in the journal *Psychogeriatrics* evaluated the effects of aromatherapy on twenty-eight elderly people suffering from dementia, with the majority also diagnosed with Alzheimer's disease. They were given rosemary and lemon inhalations in the morning, then lavender and orange in the evening. Through multiple tests and forms of analysis, the "patients showed significant improvement in personal orientation" without any deleterious side effects.[27] This study shows that orange oil—when used in combination with rosemary, lemon, and lavender—can improve cognitive ability and that it is made more powerful when part of multifunctional blends.

Application: Diffuse 3 drops each of lavender and orange essential oils at night to enjoy restful, rejuvenating sleep.

3. Relieve Anxiety

Orange oil has also been shown to help relieve presurgical anxiety in dental patients. One study looked at both orange and lavender essential oil in comparison to listening to music or no intervention. The researchers found that those patients who were exposed to the fragrance of either lavender or orange enjoyed a significant reduction in presurgical anxiety, and their mood was boosted as well.[28]

I highlight this study because these patients were battling a considerable amount of anxiety going into dental surgery. If research like this shows us how helpful orange oil (along with lavender oil) can be under stressful circumstances, imagine how it might enhance normal, everyday life!

Application: Prepare an anti-anxiety inhaler for on-the-go relief.

CITRUS LOVER'S ANXIETY INHALER

5 drops orange essential oil
5 drops bergamot essential oil
5 drops sandalwood essential oil
5 drops ylang ylang essential oil

SUPPLIES
Precut organic cotton pad
Aromatherapy inhaler

1. Place a cotton pad in the inhaler tube.
2. Drop the essential oils directly onto the cotton pad inside the tube.
3. Secure the cap and store in desk drawer, purse, or glove compartment so you have it handy.
4. When a panic attack hits or when you feel anxious, simply open the inhaler and take a few deep breaths of vapor from the tube.

4. Reduce Joint Pain

There aren't many studies on the effect of citrus oils on pain, but an interesting study from 2008 looked at the use of orange and ginger oils to reduce knee pain in a group of elderly people. Fifty-nine patients received six massage sessions over six weeks using an aromatic massage oil (1% *Zingiber officinale* and 0.5% *Citrus sinensis,* with olive oil as the carrier). Their pain started to decrease within the first week. Notably, these people regularly experienced "moderate to severe" knee pain, so the relief was most welcome. Interestingly, the pain relief wasn't permanent. It only lasted until a week after the study ended, which suggests that regular use is necessary for joint-related issues such as morning stiffness and inflammatory disease.[29]

Application: Prepare a pain relief roll-on for immediate, short-term relief.

CITRUS-POWERED PAIN RELIEF ROLL-ON

5 drops orange essential oil

5 drops copaiba essential oil

5 drops frankincense essential oil

Carrier oil of choice—jojoba and fractionated coconut oil absorb quickly and work best—as needed

SUPPLIES

10 ml glass roller bottle

1. Drop the essential oils into the roller bottle.
2. Fill the bottle with your carrier oil of choice and shake well.
3. Apply over joints during flare-ups twice daily at the onset of pain.

5. Ward Off Harmful Microbes

Like many essential oils, orange is antimicrobial. In a study of ten essential oils and their ability to kill twenty-two different strains of bacteria and twelve strains of fungi, orange oil was one of only four oils that were able to kill off all strains. The study pitted multiple types of bacteria, yeast, and fungi against essential oils, which suggests that orange can be used to treat a variety of microbial attacks.[30]

Application: Add orange to any of the DIY cleaning recipes in part 2.

A Note About d-Limonene

One of the most common terpenes in nature, d-limonene is mostly found in the rind of citrus fruits. An article in the *Alternative Medicine Review* sums up its therapeutic abilities well.[31] According to the study, d-limonene:

- "Does not pose a mutagenic, carcinogenic, or nephrotoxic risk to humans."[32]
- "Has been used clinically to dissolve cholesterol-containing gallstones."[33]
- "Has also been used for relief of heartburn and gastroesophageal reflux (GERD)."[34]
- "Has well-established chemopreventive (the ability to slow or prevent the progression of cancer) activity against many types of cancer."[35]

Additionally, we know that d-limonene is a superpower in several other ways:

- **Boosts immunity.** d-Limonene is a potent antioxidant and anti-inflammatory agent.[36]
- **Reverses liver and pancreas damage.** In an attempt to see how alternative therapies affected nonalcoholic fatty liver disease, d-limonene was shown to reverse the effects of a high-fat diet in rats and restored the damage done to their liver and pancreas.[37]
- **Kills pathogens and acts as a preservative.** Known to kill fungal threats, d-limonene can extend the shelf life of prepared foods by keeping fungal infestation and aflatoxin threats at bay.[38]
- **Aids in weight loss.** Studies on lime essential oil have uncovered its ability to not only suppress appetite, but also to promote weight loss. Researchers suggest that these properties are due to the high amounts of d-limonene found in the oil.[39]
- **Decreases stress.** As seen with bergamot oil, d-limonene has profound anti-stress effects on humans and animals.[40]

- **Promotes restful sleep.** Shown to activate adenosine A(2A) receptors, which are suspected to induce sedative effects, d-limonene can help promote a better night's sleep.[41]

ESSENTIAL OILS RICH IN D-LIMONENE

In addition to orange, dozens of other essential oils are rich sources of d-limonene.[42] Here's how they compare.

- Grapefruit (84.8%–95.4%)
- Clementine (94.8%–95.0%)
- Tangerine (87.4%–91.7%)
- Lemon, expressed (56.6%–76.0%)
- Celery seed (68.0%–75.0%)
- Mandarin (65.3%–74.2%)
- Tangelo (73.2%)
- Lemon, distilled (64.0%–70.5%)
- Dill seed (35.9%–68.4%)
- Elemi (26.9%–65.0%)
- Palo santo (58.6%–63.3%)
- Yuzu (63.1%)
- Lime, expressed (51.5%–59.6%)
- Lime, distilled (55.6%)
- Fir needle, silver (54.7%)
- Bergamot, expressed (27.4%–52.0%)
- Caraway (36.9%–48.8%)

As we have discussed before, we need to be careful about taking single chemical constituent studies out of context. Still, because they contain as much as 95% d-limonene, you can safely assume that using citrus essential oils may possibly have the same therapeutic effect as the isolated d-limonene compound itself!

READY TO TRY IT FOR YOURSELF?

Now that you've started your Essential Oils Daily Practice (from chapter 5) and you're equipped with all of the tools and tips needed to start using essential oils safely and effectively, it's time to get your hands dirty and learn how to make even more essential oil preparations!

Part 2

Dr. Z's Recommended Oils for Nearly Every Occasion

Proper planning prevents poor performance.

—BRITISH ARMY ADAGE

Once you start to incorporate essential oils into your daily routine, you'll soon realize that they offer tremendous benefit in all parts of your life—to help you manage specific illnesses and conditions, yes, but also to help you clean your home with far fewer chemicals (and far less cost) than standard cleaning supplies, to help you administer care to the pets in your life, and even to freshen up your stinky sneakers!

In the upcoming chapters, I will outline a range of basic essential oil recipes as well as show how to customize them to your desired use to benefit your body, your home, and your loved ones.

7

Basic Recipes

Once you have mastered a technique, you hardly need to look at a recipe again and can take off on your own.

—JULIA CHILD

Once you take the time to master the basic recipes that make up your favorite essential oil–based products—the carrier base, for example, or the spritzer blend—the variations you can create are limitless.

Hands down, my favorite blend of carrier oils is Mama Z's Oil Base (see page 43). I think you will love it too. But if you don't, simply try some other oils to find your own. Refer back to the list of carrier oils on page 41, and have fun experimenting.

From there, you just need to learn more about which types of oils are good for which purposes. For instance, want to promote rest and relaxation? Add a couple drops of lavender to your concoction. Want to perk up your mood? Add a citrus oil or two.

In this chapter, you'll learn these basic recipes and some general guidelines so you can start creating essential oil blends that suit you and your needs. In later chapters, we'll dive into more advanced formulas to combat specific illnesses, but for now, let's cover the fundamentals.

BASIC BATH SALTS FORMULA

Makes 1 application

1 cup Epsom salts

1 ounce unscented Dr. Bronner's liquid castile soap (acts as an emulsifier)

1 ounce carrier oil (do not use regular coconut oil, as it can harden and clog pipes)

10 drops essential oils

SUPPLIES

Medium glass bowl

1. Mix the ingredients in a bowl.

2. Pour all of the contents into the tub while drawing a bath—use the warmest water you can tolerate to fully dissolve all ingredients.

BASIC MASSAGE OIL FORMULA

Makes 1 or 2 applications

1 ounce carrier oil of your choice

12 drops essential oils

SUPPLIES

Small glass bowl

Lotion dispenser or glass jar

1. Mix the ingredients thoroughly in a bowl.

2. Use as a massage oil wherever muscles are sore. Or, to use as a moisturizer, apply to damp skin after a shower.

3. Store any leftover oil in a lotion container or glass jar.

Note: *This recipe is formulated to create a 2% dilution, which is the standard in aromatherapy for a massage oil for adults. For an exhaustive list of conversions* *that are safe for the entire family, visit chapter 2, where I discuss the topical use of essential oils and safety precautions.*

BASIC ROLLER BOTTLE FORMULA (2% DILUTION)

6 drops essential oil
Fractionated coconut oil or the carrier oil of your choice

SUPPLIES
10 ml glass roller bottle

1. Drop the essential oils into the roller bottle.
2. Fill the bottle with the carrier oil and shake gently to mix.

ROLLER BOTTLE DILUTION GUIDE

Since roller bottles usually come in 5, 10, or 15 ml bottles, the standard conversions in chapter 2 won't apply. Here is a quick roller bottle dilution guide to get you started.

	5 ML ROLLER BOTTLE (1 TEASPOON)	10 ML ROLLER BOTTLE (2 TEASPOONS)
0.5%	Less than 1 drop	1 drop
1.0%	1.5 drops	3 drops
2.0%	3 drops	6 drops
3.0%	4.5 drops	9 drops
4.0%	6 drops	12 drops
5.0%	7.5 drops	15 drops

BASIC DIFFUSER FORMULA

5 drops essential oils per 150 ml water

SUPPLIES
Diffuser

1. Fill the diffuser with water to the predetermined line (usually 150 ml).
2. Add the essential oils.
3. Run the diffuser in a well-ventilated room until the water is used up.

Note: *Clean the diffuser with a dry paper towel before your next use.*

BASIC SPRITZER FORMULA

10 drops organic grain alcohol (190 proof) per 1 ounce distilled water
10 drops essential oils per 1 ounce distilled water
10 drops witch hazel per 1 ounce distilled water

SUPPLIES
1- or 2-ounce spray bottle

1. Mix the grain alcohol, essential oils, and witch hazel in the bottle.
2. Add distilled water and shake vigorously.

Note: *This formula will last for a couple of weeks. I've had these last for as long as two months and have not noticed any bacterial overgrowth, which can happen with all water-based products. This may not be obvious at first, but the smell will become rancid and you will notice a change in color if it is contaminated.*

BASIC CAPSULE FORMULA

Makes 1 dose

4 drops essential oils
Organic, unrefined coconut oil or olive oil

SUPPLIES
Pipette
Size 00 time-release capsule

1. Using a pipette, drop the essential oils into the narrower bottom half of the capsule.

2. Use the pipette to fill the remaining space in the capsule with coconut or olive oil.

3. Fit the wider top half of the capsule over the bottom half and secure snugly.

4. Swallow a capsule immediately with water on an empty stomach. Take twice daily.

Note: *Do not premake and store for future use.*

LET'S GET STARTED

Now that we've covered some basic formulas, I recommend starting with Mama Z's Healing Skin Serum, which you can find at the end of this chapter. A little more advanced, it will help lay the foundation for many more recipes to come as it facilitates healing at the deepest levels and can be used for a wide variety of skin conditions.

The story behind this formulation tells how my wife helped her father beat skin cancer. My hope and prayer is that it inspires you to make your own and even give some away to a loved one who may be in need.

MAMA Z'S STORY

My dad is a retired agriscientist and he has always been—and likely always will be—a passionate hobby farmer. In addition to his full-time job, he has spent more than forty hours per week in the garden for as long as I can remember. He lived outside during the growing season any time he wasn't at work, and a lot of our family time was spent picking weeds and harvesting our produce. Even now, long retired from the agriculture business, he's still in the garden year-round. I have him to thank for my work ethic, my green thumb, and my sensitive skin!

Dad's been bald for many years now and he's always had a problem with cancerous lesions on his scalp. He goes through ball caps like my mom and I go through panty hose, but that still doesn't keep all the sun away from his pale, Irish/Scandinavian skin. For decades, my dad has battled melanoma on his head and has also recently developed precancerous lesions on his arms and hands.

During my dad's most recent bout with skin cancer, he showed me the cream his doctor prescribed. One of its side effects was cancer! Isn't that crazy?? I still can't get over the insanity behind an anti–skin cancer cream that can cause cancer in other parts of the body.

Dad had been applying this cream on his skin for months after having several tumors removed. Unfortunately, this approach didn't really help at all. In fact, the skin began to scale and resembled a candida infection.

I asked him if he wanted to be healed and he said, "Of course!" I asked him if he'd be willing to try my favorite DIY anti-aging skin cream and he said yes, but only if he could finish off the prescription stuff he was using. I said, "Fair enough," and went to work.

I ended up making my dad two varieties of my anti-aging cream for him to try: one with lavender oil only and another with a blend of lavender, tea tree, and frankincense. He used both my cream and the prescription stuff for a short time and ended up using my concoctions alone. From what we can tell, the precancerous lesions were not a sign of a candida infection and they simply disappeared and didn't progress to melanoma.

Within six weeks, his hands and arms were completely clear, and now he's a believer in the power of DIY with essential oils!

MAMA Z'S HEALING SKIN SERUM

This supereasy serum can be used as a carrier for any of your favorite essential oils. It is very good for the skin on its own, but even better with essential oils!

4 ounces aloe vera gel

4 ounces organic, unrefined coconut oil (melted)

32 drops lavender essential oil

16 drops frankincense essential oil (any species will do)

16 drops tea tree essential oil

8 drops sandalwood essential oil

SUPPLIES

Food processer or blender

Glass storage container

1. Blend the aloe gel, coconut oil, and essential oils in a food processor or blender until smooth.

2. Once well mixed, store in a glass jar or salve container in a cool place (like the fridge) so the coconut oil remains hardened.

3. Apply over any problem areas on your skin at least once per day.

➔ To watch me and Mama Z make her Healing Skin Serum go to HealingPowerOfEssentialOils.com.

The reviews we've received from our online fans about this serum are pretty fantastic. They're using it to treat everything from psoriasis to dermatitis to sunburns. Try it out and let me know what you think by leaving a comment on my website. I'd love to hear from you!

8

Heal Yourself

Fruit trees of all kinds will grow on both banks of the river. Their leaves will not wither, nor will their fruit fail. Every month they will bear fruit, because the water from the sanctuary flows to them. Their fruit will serve for food and their leaves for healing.

—EZEKIEL 47:12

Bits and pieces of my personal healing story have been shared with millions of people around the globe. Like so many whom I have been privileged to help over the years, I suffered because I was a victim of misinformation. The more I studied biblical health and researched what the medical literature had to say about staying well and preventing disease, the more I encountered the notion that focusing on gut health should be the top priority.

While you traverse your own health journey, my recommendation is that you take a good look at your gut first, because it is the cornerstone of your health. And it's why I begin our medicine cabinet makeover by focusing on the gastrointestinal tract!

DR. Z'S MEDICINE CABINET MAKEOVER

In this section, I cover effective remedies for the following five conditions:

1. Gastrointestinal Health
- Oral health
- Stomach and digestive health
- Gut health

2. Mental Health
- Energy and focus
- Mood enhancement
- Stress

3. Infections
- Immune-boosting
- General infection protocol (specific infections like candida are discussed in later chapters)

4. Pain Management
- General pain
- Headaches and migraines
- Hemorrhoids

5. Sleep and Weight Loss
- Relaxing into sleep
- Appetite suppression
- Fat burning

GASTROINTESTINAL HEALTH

The gastrointestinal (GI) tract connects your mouth to your anus, and every part in between is important and cannot be overlooked. I will discuss below some essential oil remedies for the three most important areas—oral health, stomach and digestive health, and gut health.

Gut health is absolutely critical to enjoying full health and wellness in body and mind, but treating the gut can be tricky. To ensure that essential oils are able to bypass gastric juices and reach the gut, you must consume them within enteric-coated capsules (also known as time-release capsules), which are manufactured with a polymer coating that is designed to be broken down in the intestines. However, you can't always find them on Amazon and often have to purchase them in bulk.

I also recommend applying a blend of gut-healing oils over the abdomen to treat digestive and gut-related concerns. Although the efficacy of this treatment has not been proven, I have seen many individuals experience amazing results. I suspect this is the case because oils applied on the skin get absorbed into the bloodstream.

Treating the oral cavity and stomach is much easier and can be accomplished by applying essential oils directly into your mouth or consuming them in regular, store-bought gel capsules to reach the stomach.

Oral Health

First on our GI health journey is oral health, where it all starts. Without question, oil pulling a few times a week is the most effective way to prevent oral health problems. When you add essential oils like clove and peppermint to your oil-pulling regimen, you experience even greater benefits. You can learn more about oil pulling with essential oils in chapter 2.

In my opinion the three most effective essential oils for oral health are clove, orange, and peppermint. Here's a quick rundown on how you can use them.

- **Canker sores.** Apply a 25% blend of my Immunity-Boosting Blend (cinnamon bark, cinnamon leaf, clove, frankincense, lemon, orange, and rosemary) with fractionated coconut oil directly on top of canker sores twice daily.
- **Halitosis.** Make the DIY toothpaste and mouthwash recipes in chapter 9 and use daily.
- **Sensitive teeth.** Oil pulling with clove is great for sensitive teeth. For extra support, apply a 50% blend of clove or orange oil with fractionated coconut oil directly on top of the teeth and gums where you're having a problem.
- **Plaque and stains.** Cinnamon leaf, clove, eucalyptus, rosemary, and orange are great to whiten teeth and clean plaque. I like to alternate these oils or blend them together and create a healthy oral mixture by adding them to my DIY toothpaste at a maximum 1% dilution.
- **Blood blisters.** Apply a 25% blend of lavender with fractionated coconut oil directly on top of blood blisters twice daily.

Stomach and Digestive Health

As we travel down the GI tract, next is the stomach and digestive health as a whole. Essential oils can help you with many common digestive ailments, including:

- **Nausea.** Simply smelling lemon oil from a bottle can stop nausea in its tracks. Same with diffusing ginger. Alternatively, taking 2 or 3 drops of a blend of peppermint, ginger, and cardamom internally in a gel capsule can help as well. Be sure to fill up your capsule with an edible carrier oil to help ensure safety and efficacy.
- **Gas and bloating.** Applying a 3%–5% dilution of my Healthy Digestion Blend (see chapter 2) over your tummy can do wonders to keep gas and bloating at bay.
- **Ulcers.** The gastroprotective abilities of clove essential oil and its primary constituent, eugenol, have been evaluated for their antiulcer activity in animal models, and both were shown to help considerably.[1] Similar effects were seen with ginger and turmeric essential oils.[2] To enjoy the ulcer-preventing prowess of clove and eugenol-containing oils, such as cinnamon (from the bark or the leaf), basil, bay laurel, and holy basil, try putting 2 drops in a size 00 gel capsule mixed with a cooking oil like coconut or olive and consume twice daily.

Gut Health

Traveling even farther down the GI tract we get to the gut, which is not only responsible for digestion and elimination, but also plays a huge role in immunity and mental health. Essential oils support good gut health in the following ways:

Irritable bowel syndrome (IBS)

IBS affects more than 10 percent of the global population, but fewer than 30 percent of those affected will ever go to the doctor to seek a diagnosis.[3] IBS is usually managed with diet and medication, but essential oils—especially in enteric-coated capsules—have also been indicated for symptom control.

Although more extensive studies are welcomed, a comprehensive review conducted in 2008 shows that peppermint oil offers significant improvement over a placebo, as does dietary fiber—both are about as effective as antispasmodic medications.[4]

Application: To ensure the oil reaches the intestines, use enteric-coated capsules. Try using 3 drops of peppermint with an edible carrier oil twice a day for a week to see how your body responds.

Dysbiosis and small intestine bacterial overgrowth (SIBO)

The microbial balance in the gut can be shifted in many ways, usually categorized as dysbiosis. A particularly concerning form of dysbiosis is SIBO, which occurs when bacteria that should be in the colon are found in the small intestine. Both generalized dysbiosis and the more specific condition of SIBO are connected to other health concerns, including IBS and metabolic disorders.[5]

A 2012 study found that specific essential oils can be paired with probiotics to relieve the symptoms of SIBO and other gut flora issues.[6] In another study, caraway, lavender, and neroli were among eight standout examples of essential oils that helped promote the balance of beneficial bacteria in the body.[7] These studies demonstrate the excellent ability of these essential oils to reduce detrimental bacteria without also lowering the population of beneficial strains.

Application: Create a SIBO blend by mixing a 1:1:1 ratio of caraway, lavender, and neroli. Then consume 2 or 3 drops of this blend in an enteric-coated capsule filled with an edible carrier oil twice a day and see how your body responds.

Leaky gut

Still a relatively new topic in the essential oil research community, leaky gut ("intestinal permeability") refers to the integrity of the intestinal barrier known as tight junctions. When the tight junctions in your intestinal lining break down or separate slightly (imagine a dam that has holes in it and leaks water), contents in the gut start to permeate the bloodstream. These toxins, proteins, and semidigested food particles are normally excreted when the system is functioning properly. The result is quite detrimental because of the ensuing inflammatory response, which can play a role in autoimmune disease, Celiac disease, IBS, mood disorders, food allergies and sensitivities, and obesity.[8]

In 2016, the *BioMed Research International* journal published a study that uncovered oregano oil's ability to repair the intestinal lining and potentially reverse leaky gut. It can close the dam, so to speak (filling in the leaky part of the gut).[9] In this particular study, the blood toxin levels from the pigs being tested decreased significantly—a good sign that ingesting oregano can help prevent toxic leakage through your gut as well.

Application: Try taking 2 or 3 drops of oregano oil in an enteric-coated capsule twice a day for a week to see if your symptoms of leaky gut subside. Be sure to fill up your capsule with an edible carrier oil to help ensure safety and efficacy.

MENTAL HEALTH

Although there are certainly times when working with a certified counselor or even taking a prescription medication can make all the difference in your mental health, essential oils can support mental health in a variety of ways, from promoting focus to reducing stress and anxiety and improving mood.

Focus and clarity

Essential oils can help you focus on what's important and think clearly—two crucial skills for keeping your thoughts trained on the positive and warding off the doubts and fears that derail so many good intentions.

When you need help pulling yourself out of a Facebook wormhole so you can get back on task, a blend of eucalyptus, peppermint, and rosemary oils can help you "be here now."

ENERGY AND FOCUS INHALER

4 drops eucalyptus essential oil

4 drops frankincense essential oil

4 drops peppermint essential oil

4 drops rosemary essential oil

4 drops sandalwood essential oil

SUPPLIES

Precut organic cotton pad

Aromatherapy inhaler

1. Place a cotton pad in the inhaler tube.

2. Drop the essential oils directly onto the cotton pad inside the tube.

3. Open the inhaler and take five deep breaths when you need a quick, focused boost of energy and mental clarity.

Mood enhancement, anxiety, and stress reduction

Essential oils are often used for their uplifting, antidepressant abilities thanks to their simple applications and quick results. It never ceases to amaze me that simply smelling a fragrance can so quickly and effectively reach and affect the brain!

There is an abundance of research showing how essential oils can enhance mood and reduce anxiety and stress. Here are just a few of those oils:

- Bergamot[10]
- Frankincense[11]
- Geranium[12]
- German chamomile[13]
- Lavender[14]
- Lemon[15]
- Neroli[16]
- Orange, sweet[17]
- Palmarosa[18]
- Peppermint[19]
- Rose[20]
- Spikenard[21]
- Ylang ylang[22]

Below are a stress-reducing blend and a mood-boosting blend that are hands down my favorites for keeping the heart light and spirits high.

DR. Z'S STRESS BOMB BLEND

20 drops frankincense essential oil

20 drops lavender essential oil

20 drops palmarosa essential oil

10 drops spikenard essential oil

10 drops ylang ylang essential oil

SUPPLIES
Small glass bottle or jar

1. Combine the essential oils in a bottle or jar and shake to mix well.
2. Use in an inhaler, diffuser, or in your DIY body oil to stop stress in its tracks!

MOOD-BOOSTING INHALER

10 drops bergamot essential oil

10 drops key lime essential oil

SUPPLIES
Precut organic cotton pad
Aromatherapy inhaler

1. Place a cotton pad in the inhaler tube.
2. Drop the essential oils directly onto the cotton pad inside the tube.
3. Open the inhaler and take five deep breaths when you feel stressed and need a pick-me-up.

Note: *Sweet or wild orange, neroli, lemon, or tangerine can be used instead of key lime if you don't have this oil.*

INFECTIONS

Infections thrive in dysfunctional immune systems. Environmental toxins abound and it's virtually impossible to find pure air, food, and water—which contributes to the gradual, systematic breakdown of our immune systems. If we regularly focus on healthy living practices, we can combat some of the effects of these toxins on our bodies.

Frankincense is the star player of the essential oils team when it comes to boosting the immune system. Research has shown that it can increase production of key components of the immune system, including cytokines (signaling molecules) and immunoglobulins (antibodies), as well as improving the function of T cells (molecules that fight invaders).

In addition to frankincense, there are other essential oils that pack a superpowerful immune system boost. To cover your bases, I suggest making an immunity-boosting blend like the one in chapter 2 with cinnamon bark, cinnamon leaf, clove, frankincense, lemon, sweet or wild orange, and rosemary.

Application: Try my Immune Booster to beef up your immune system.

IMMUNE BOOSTER

1 packet liposomal vitamin C (preferably LivOn Labs brand)
1 teaspoon raw honey
1 teaspoon organic, unrefined coconut oil
1 or 2 drops Immunity-Boosting Blend (page 50)
¼ teaspoon organic pumpkin pie spice
Tiny pinch of Himalayan pink sea salt
Warm water, as needed

SUPPLIES
Medium drinking glass

1. Mix all the ingredients in a glass, then dilute with warm water to taste.
2. Enjoy twice daily at the onset of a cold, or once per day for prevention during cold and flu season.

Note: *This is not a long-term solution, and using for more than two or three weeks at a time is not advisable. Be sure to consult with your health care provider if you're* *currently taking immune-suppressing medications for an autoimmune condition. Discontinue the blend if adverse reactions occur.*

MULTIPURPOSE INFECTION-FIGHTING ROLL-ON

If you find yourself with a weakened immune system and you come down with an infection (bacterial, fungal, or viral), try this multipurpose roll-on.

2 drops lemongrass essential oil
2 drops sweet or wild orange essential oil
2 drops oregano essential oil
2 drops tea tree essential oil
2 drops thyme essential oil
Fractionated coconut oil (almond or jojoba can also be used)

SUPPLIES
10 ml glass roller bottle

1. Mix the essential oils in the roller bottle.
2. Fill with the coconut oil and gently shake to mix.
3. Apply on the soles of the feet and over the abdomen twice a day while battling a systemic infection.

Note: *Do not use for more than three weeks at a time. Discontinue use immediately if you experience any adverse reactions. Also, do not use on an open wound. For that purpose, apply a 3% dilution of lavender oil topically every 4 hours (3% = 18 drops per ounce of an antifungal carrier oil such as unrefined coconut oil).*

GENERAL PAIN CONDITIONS

Peppermint oil and lavender oil work well together as a cooling, soothing anti-inflammatory for painful areas. Lemon balm (*Melissa*) essential oil has also been shown to have some effectiveness against both inflammation and swelling.[23]

Application: Whip up one of the following blends in a carrier oil and you'll have a healthier bottle of relief to reach for the next time you're in pain.

PAIN AWAY BODY OIL

10 drops lavender essential oil
10 drops peppermint essential oil
5 drops lemon balm essential oil
1 ounce carrier oil (we use Mama Z's Oil Base, page 43)

SUPPLIES
Glass jar

1. Drop the essential oils into the glass jar.
2. Add the carrier oil and mix.
3. Massage over painful joints or into sore muscles as needed.

For deeper relief, you might need to up the ante; frankincense can help. The pain-relieving ability of this essential oil was tested on patients struggling with cancer, who were either treated to a week of daily five-minute hand massages with sweet almond oil infused with essential oils of bergamot, lavender, and frankincense in a 1:1:1 ratio in a 1.5% dilution, or a week of daily five-minute hand massages with sweet almond oil that had no essential oils. With no other pain medications used, the group who received the essential oil massage with frankincense reported that their pain was relieved significantly.[24] Because there is a connection between inflammatory processes and pain, oils that are anti-inflammatory are often analgesic as well. Frankincense serves this dual role.

Other oils that are especially helpful in combating serious pain conditions are copaiba (*Copaifera langsdorffii*) and sweet marjoram (*Origanum majorana*).[25]

Application: Try my No More Pain Blend for deep relief.

NO MORE PAIN BLEND

25 drops copaiba essential oil
25 drops frankincense essential oil
25 drops sweet marjoram essential oil

SUPPLIES
5 ml essential oil bottle

1. Mix the essential oils in a 5 ml bottle.
2. Use as directed in the following recipes.

NO MORE PAIN ROLL-ON

15 drops No More Pain Blend
Fractionated coconut oil

SUPPLIES
10 ml glass roller bottle

1. Drop the essential oils into the roller bottle.
2. Fill the roller bottle with your carrier oil of choice (fractionated coconut oil works best) and shake well.
3. Massage over sore muscles and joints. Wait 4 hours between applications.

NO MORE PAIN CAPSULES

Makes 1 application

2 or 3 drops No More Pain Blend
Olive oil

SUPPLIES
Pipette
Size 00 gel capsule

1. With a pipette, put 2 or 3 drops of the No More Pain Blend into a gel capsule and fill with olive oil.
2. Take up to twice a day as needed.

Note: *This is not a long-term solution, and using for more than two or three weeks at a time is not advisable. Be sure to consult with your health care provider first if you're currently taking medications. Discontinue if adverse reactions occur.*

Headaches and Migraines

You can enjoy great relief from headaches and migraines by using essential oils. The spicy tingle of peppermint oil helps relieve the muscular tension that leads to headache and, when blended with lavender and wintergreen, can be highly effective at stopping an attack.

INSTANT HEADACHE AND MIGRAINE RELIEF

7 drops peppermint essential oil
7 drops lavender essential oil
2 drops copaiba essential oil
2 drops frankincense essential oil
2 drops wintergreen essential oil
1 ounce carrier oil or Mama Z's Oil Base (page 43)

SUPPLIES
Small glass bowl
Glass jar or bottle

1. Drop the essential oils into the bowl.
2. Add the carrier oil and mix.
3. Massage over the temples and back of the neck at the onset of a headache or migraine.
4. Store the excess in a glass jar.

Hemorrhoids

Hemorrhoids are usually caused by excessive straining to make a bowel movement. Essential oils won't prevent them; however, they can significantly reduce the discomfort as your body heals (eating a healthy, fiber- and probiotic-rich diet will also help prevent them from happening in the first place). Traditionally thought to help constrict blood vessels that can cause a hemorrhoid to swell, cypress oil (*Cupressus sempervirens*) is a key ingredient in the following DIY recipes.

HEMORRHOID SITZ BATH

1 cup Epsom salts

1 ounce evening primrose oil

1 ounce jojoba oil

1 ounce Dr. Bronner's unscented liquid castile soap

1 drop cypress essential oil

1 drop frankincense essential oil

1 drop lavender essential oil

1 drop Roman chamomile essential oil

Hot water, as needed

SUPPLIES

Large glass bowl

1. Put the Epsom salts in the bowl, add the carrier oils and castile soap, and mix until evenly distributed.
2. Add the essential oils and mix well.
3. Pour in just enough hot water to dissolve the salts.
4. Fill a tub with 4 or 5 inches of warm water, making sure it's not too hot for your bottom.
5. Add the Epsom salts and oil mixture.
6. Sit down in the bath so that your bottom is immersed in the mixture and soak for 15 to 20 minutes.
7. Rinse both yourself and the tub afterward.

HEMORRHOID CREAM

2 ounces Mama Z's Oil Base (page 43)
15 drops cypress essential oil
10 drops peppermint essential oil
5 drops frankincense essential oil
5 drops lavender essential oil

SUPPLIES
Small glass jar

1. Mix the ingredients in a small jar, secure the lid, and refrigerate until hardened.
2. After washing your hands, carefully apply a small dab directly onto your hemorrhoid twice daily to calm the inflammation and soothe the pain.
3. Store extra in the refrigerator.

SLEEP AND WEIGHT LOSS

The sleep aid and weight loss markets are big money, which presents a huge problem for those of us in the public health world because the products being recommended are often habit forming. This is also why I clump sleep and weight loss together—because medicine cabinets across the land are filled with addictive and mostly useless over-the-counter pills that do not truly address the issues behind insomnia and unwanted weight gain.

Lavender is a superstar when it comes to promoting sleep—it is found in the vast majority of studies that evaluate essential oils for sleep relief. Using lavender oil as a sleep aid can be as simple as inhaling its scent straight out of the bottle! If you'd like a more formal recipe, try one of the following blends.

SLEEPY-TIME SPRITZ

20 drops Sleepy-Time Blend (page 50)
20 drops organic grain alcohol (190 proof)
20 drops witch hazel

2-ounce glass spray bottle

1. Combine the essential oils, grain alcohol, and witch hazel in the spray bottle and gently shake to mix.
2. Fill the remaining space in the bottle with water and shake well.
3. Mist your pillow before bedtime to help aid sleep and provide a restful night.

SWEET SLUMBER DIFFUSER BLEND

5 drops of your favorite sleep-inducing blend (see the box below for ideas)

SUPPLIES

Diffuser

1. Fill the diffuser with water as directed.
2. Add the essential oils.
3. Start the diffuser 10 minutes before you get into bed.

ESSENTIAL OIL BLENDS FOR SLEEP

In addition to the Sleepy-Time Blend on page 50, these are some of my favorite and most-used blends for a restful night's sleep:

- Frankincense, myrrh, and vetiver
- Cedarwood, sandalwood, and valerian
- Clary sage, lavender, sweet marjoram, rose-scented geranium, and ylang ylang
- Sweet or wild orange, palmarosa, and patchouli

In addition to putting these oils in your diffuser, you can add 5 drops of an oil blend to ½ cup white vinegar and put it in the fabric softener cup of your washing machine when you wash your sheets. Or, drop the oils on a wet washcloth and toss it in the dryer when you dry your sheets.

SWEET SLEEP BODY OIL

4 drops lavender essential oil

4 drops Roman chamomile essential oil

4 drops vetiver essential oil

4 drops ylang ylang essential oil

2 ounces carrier oil or Mama Z's Oil Base (page 43)

SUPPLIES

Medium glass bowl

Lotion dispenser or glass jar

1. Drop the essential oils into the bowl.
2. Add a carrier oil and mix.
3. Use to massage your feet and as a body oil before bedtime for added moisture and supersweet sleep.
4. Store the excess in a lotion dispenser or glass jar.

➡ To watch me and Mama Z make Sweet Sleep Body Oil and learn how our family of six enjoys great sleep every night, go to HealingPowerOfEssentialOils.com.

Weight Loss

To use essential oils to lose weight, research has suggested that lime (*Citrus aurantifolia*) is your best bet, primarily because of its ability to naturally suppress appetite.[26] Another study found that women who massaged their abdomen twice a day for six weeks using a 3% solution of grapefruit and cypress oils experienced a significant decrease in abdominal fat and waist circumference. As an added bonus, the women who used the essential oil treatment reported a notable improvement in body image.[27]

This Fat-Burning Roll-On incorporates these two oils, and is an adaptation of what Mama Z used to help her trim down and burn fat for the 2017 Mrs. Georgia pageant.

FAT-BURNING ROLL-ON

4 drops lime essential oil

3 drops peppermint essential oil

3 drops grapefruit essential oil

2 drops cypress essential oil

1 drop eucalyptus essential oil

1 drop cinnamon bark essential oil

Enough of your favorite carrier oil to fill the roller bottle—fractionated coconut oil, jojoba, or sweet almond all work great!

SUPPLIES

10 ml glass roller bottle

1. Drop the essential oils into the bottle.
2. Fill the bottle with your favorite carrier oil.
3. Mix by shaking vigorously for 10 seconds.
4. Apply over problem areas like the stomach, back of the thighs, and undersides of the upper arms after your shower 3 or 4 times per week.

Note: *Test a skin patch first on the back of your hand or bottoms of the feet to make sure your body responds well to the blend. Discontinue use immediately if irritation occurs.*

FAT-BURNING WRAP

Wrapping the part of your body you're seeking to slim down after you've applied the Fat-Burning Roll-On will help increase absorption and prevent your sheets and clothes from absorbing the oils instead of your skin. Works great on the back of the legs to minimize cellulite!

Fat-Burning Roll-On, as needed

SUPPLIES
1 yard of muslin fabric, cut into strips large enough to cover the body part you want to treat but small enough to be manageable
Plastic wrap

1. Right before bed, liberally apply the Fat-Burning Roll-On over areas of concern.
2. Wrap each area of the body individually with muslin.
3. Wrap the fabric with two or three layers of plastic wrap.
4. When you wake up, unwrap each area and wipe yourself down with a towel before showering.

9

Personal Care Products

My people are destroyed for lack of knowledge.

—HOSEA 4:6

When she was fourteen years old, Mama Z went to visit her grandparents in Minnesota. Preparing for the trip, she went to K-Mart, purchased two conventional facial cleansers, and didn't think twice about it. When she arrived at her grandparents' home, she went to wash her face. And something horrific happened.

The chemicals in the well water interacted with the chemicals in the facial cleansers and literally burned off the first few layers of Mama Z's skin from her nose to her neck. The pain was excruciating and she was devastated when she looked into the mirror. Oozing sores peppered her face, causing physical and emotional pain. To make matters worse, nothing she did seemed to help.

It wasn't until she consulted her mom's close friend, Mrs. B, a Native American from the Cherokee tribe who practices Ojibwe medicine, that things started to turn around.

Mrs. B told Sabrina to use a homemade cream including lavender oil and blessed her with an essential oils starter kit. Within a couple of weeks, Sabrina's skin completely healed up and even today, you won't find any scars.

Teenage Mama Z fell into a trap that millions of people fall into every day: believing that the Food and Drug Administration (FDA) approves only healthy products for us to use, and that manufacturers do their best to sell only good stuff. Nothing could be further from the truth. Don't forget that the health and beauty market is *big* business, and many companies will do whatever it takes to save money, even if this involves using additives, fillers, and preservatives that are not safe to apply to the human body! The lengthy lineup of uncertain ingredients can be eye-opening because it doesn't seem to end, as new chemicals are introduced nearly every day.

As health and beauty manufacturers rake in the dough, we are playing Russian roulette by using products with questionable ingredients that could very well trigger myriad health conditions. This is a very serious public health concern that has further-reaching effects than you might think. Take the landmark Environmental Working Group (EWG) study from 2005. Until relatively recently, scientists thought that the human placenta protected the baby from external toxins. In a research trial evaluating the cord blood of a random sample of ten babies born in the United States during August and September of 2004, researchers at two independent laboratories uncovered that up to a total of 287 industrial chemicals and pollutants could be found in the infants' umbilical cord blood, including consumer product ingredients, pesticides, and wastes from burning coal, gasoline, and garbage![1]

According to the study, "Of the 287 chemicals we detected in umbilical cord blood, we know that 180 cause cancer in humans or animals, 217 are toxic to the brain and nervous system, and 208 cause birth defects or abnormal development in animal tests. The dangers of pre- or post-natal exposure to this complex mixture of carcinogens, developmental toxins and neurotoxins have never been studied."[2]

YOUR ALLY IN FINDING SAFE PERSONAL CARE PRODUCTS

The EWG has become my go-to resource to determine if the store-bought body care items we use at home are safe. You can investigate yours as well by checking out the massive Skin Deep Database at www.EWG.org/SkinDeep, where EWG lists the ingredients and potential toxic exposure of more than sixty-five thousand body care items on the market today.

Despite the thoroughness of EWG's database, the only way to truly ensure that you're not inadvertently harming yourself and your family is by making personal care products yourself. And the first place to start is with antibacterial products.

CASE IN POINT: THE BANNING OF TRICLOSAN

In September 2016, the FDA finally issued a ruling that officially banned the use of triclocarban, triclosan, and seventeen other dangerous chemicals in hand and body washes. These products have been marketed as being more effective than good old-fashioned soap and water and consumers have been misled into purchasing them.[3]

"Consumers may think antibacterial washes are more effective at preventing the spread of germs, but we have no scientific evidence that they are any better than plain soap and water," stated Janet Woodcock, MD, director of the FDA's Center for Drug Evaluation and Research. "In fact, some data suggests that antibacterial ingredients may do more harm than good over the long term."[4]

Antibacterial product manufacturers were given one year to comply with the new law by removing all products from the market that violate this ruling. But this still isn't enough to keep us safe. Triclosan is still in countless other products like deodorants, antiperspirants, body spray, and toothpastes!

Triclosan-laden antibacterial products kill all the bacteria on your hands, including the *good* bacteria you need for healthy skin and a properly functioning immune system. In fact, these products have been shown to weaken your immune system![5]

ELIMINATE TOXIC BODY CARE PRODUCTS BY MAKING THEM YOURSELF

The solution is simple: Toss all those antibacterial products in the trash and start to make your own. I've created recipes for all of the basic products you need to get started.

HAND SANITIZER SPRAY

Organic grain alcohol (190 proof)
Distilled water
15 drops Immunity-Boosting Blend (page 50) or other oil(s) you prefer
2 or 3 drops vitamin E (optional)
2 or 3 drops aloe (optional)

SUPPLIES
1-ounce glass spray bottle

1. Fill a quarter of the bottle with grain alcohol and the rest with water.
2. Choose the essential oils to add that meet your desired result—for example, if you want a soothing sanitizer, use lavender; if you want an uplifting blend, use sweet or wild orange.
3. If you want a moisturizing spray, add some vitamin E and aloe.
4. Shake to blend.
5. Spray on your hands and rub them together as you would with a conventional hand sanitizer.

POPULAR ESSENTIAL OILS FOR SOAP

- Geranium and lavender
- Lemon, lime, or grapefruit
- Eucalyptus and tea tree
- Immunity-Boosting Blend (page 50)

HEALTHY BACTERIA LIQUID HAND SOAP

This hand soap targets only pathogenic microorganisms, helping to ensure that the healthy bacteria remain on your skin.

¼ cup distilled water
¼ cup Dr. Bronner's liquid castile soap

1½ teaspoons vitamin E oil
1½ teaspoons sweet almond or jojoba oil
20 drops of the essential oil or blend of your choice

SUPPLIES
Glass bottle with pump or glass foaming soap dispenser

1. In glass bottle combine the water and liquid soap.
2. Add your vitamin E, sweet almond or jojoba oil, and essential oils.
3. Screw on the lid and shake well.

Note: *If you make this soap in a larger amount, store the leftovers in a glass jar until your containers need a refill; just remember to always shake well before using.*

FOAMING HAND SOAP

This alternative is just as effective as the liquid hand soap and even easier to make! The exact measurements depend on the size of your foaming soap dispenser.

Dr. Bronner's liquid castile soap
Aloe vera gel
Essential oils

SUPPLIES
Glass foaming soap dispenser or foaming soap pump to use with mason jar

1. Fill your soap dispenser three-fifths of the way with liquid soap.
2. Add enough aloe to fill the dispenser four-fifths of the way. (Be sure to leave enough room in the bottle to place the pump without overflowing.)
3. Top it off with essential oils (10 drops for every ounce of your mixture).
4. Depending on the thickness of the aloe vera, you may need to add a little water. The consistency should feel like that of a traditional pump soap.
5. Secure the pump and shake vigorously.

EXFOLIATING CITRUS SUGAR SCRUB FOR BODY

Cleanse away dead skin without worrying about rubbing toxic chemicals into your skin. (But avoid using on face as it is too abrasive for the delicate skin there.)

6 tablespoons organic Fair Trade sugar

4 teaspoons carrier oil

¼ cup raw local honey

5 drops bergamot essential oil

5 drops grapefruit essential oil

5 drops lime or lemon essential oil

SUPPLIES

Small glass bowl

Glass jar or bottle for storage

1. Mix all the ingredients in the bowl.
2. Store in a glass container.
3. Use 1 to 2 tablespoons as desired as an exfoliating scrub in the bath or shower.

ESSENTIAL OILS FOR HAIR CARE

- For all hair types: rosemary, sage, or rose
- For oily hair: lemon, bergamot, or tea tree
- For dry hair or to treat dandruff: lavender, sandalwood, or geranium
- To stimulate growth: peppermint or rosemary

REJUVENATING SHAMPOO

You're going to love the essential oil–based versions of these classic shampoo and conditioner DIY recipes.

1 cup Dr. Bronner's liquid castile soap

½ cup full-fat coconut milk

1 tablespoon aloe vera gel

1 teaspoon carrier oil

25 drops essential oils (from the list of essential oils for hair care on page 146)

5 drops carrot seed oil

5 drops red raspberry seed oil (optional for color-treated hair)

SUPPLIES

Immersion or regular blender

Glass bowl or jar for mixing

Glass pump bottle for storage and dispensing

1. Combine all ingredients in a blender or glass bowl or jar.

2. Blend well using an immersion blender or a regular blender, or by vigorously shaking a glass jar.

3. Pour the shampoo into a glass pump bottle for easy dispensing and storage.

REJUVENATING CONDITIONER

1 teaspoon carrier oil of your choice

2 teaspoons guar gum

25 drops essential oils (from the list of essential oils for hair care on page 146)

1 teaspoon aloe vera gel

5 drops carrot seed oil

5 drops red raspberry seed oil (optional for color-treated hair)

1 cup distilled water

SUPPLIES

Glass pump bottle

1. In a glass pump bottle, mix the carrier oil, guar gum, essential oils, aloe vera gel, carrot seed oil, and red raspberry seed oil.

2. Add the distilled water and shake well.

Note: *Guar gum is a natural thickener often used in baking and cosmetics, often available in the baking section of the grocery store—Bob's Red Mill is a popular brand.*

PURE AIR HAIR SPRAY

You don't have to hold your breath while using this toxin-free hair spray!

1 cup distilled water
1 tablespoon organic, Fair Trade granulated sugar or coconut sugar
25 drops essential oils (see Note)

SUPPLIES
Small saucepan
Whisk
Glass spray misting bottle

1. Bring the water to a simmer, then remove from heat.
2. Add the sugar and whisk until completely dissolved.
3. Allow the mixture to cool before adding the essential oils.
4. Store in a glass spray bottle with a fine mister.
5. Shake before each use to distribute the oils, as they will separate.

Note: *Many essential oils can increase your photosensitivity, so they should be used with caution. If you plan on spending all day in the sun, you shouldn't use the potentially phototoxic oils listed in chapter 2 (page 54) as the skin on your scalp can get sunburned, particularly if you are balding or have thinning hair.*

SAMPLE ESSENTIAL OIL BLENDS FOR ORAL CARE

- Bergamot, lemon, grapefruit
- Sweet or wild orange, clove, peppermint, spearmint
- Cinnamon bark or cinnamon leaf, clove, sweet or wild orange
- Roman chamomile, spearmint, wintergreen
- Frankincense, lime, myrrh

REMINERALIZING TOOTH POWDER

Before there was toothpaste as we know it today, people used tooth powder to help clean their teeth. Sprinkled (rather than squeezed) on your toothbrush, tooth powder is simply a less spreadable form of toothpaste. If you prefer a more traditional toothpaste, you can add coconut oil to this mixture (see Note).

10 drops essential oils (from the list of essential oil blends for oral care on page 148)
¼ cup hot distilled water
1 tablespoon coconut oil (more if making toothpaste)
⅓ cup bentonite clay
1½ teaspoons stevia powder
¼ teaspoon Himalayan pink sea salt

SUPPLIES
Small glass bowl
Medium glass bowl for mixing
Food processor
Small glass jar for storing

1. Mix your essential oils in a small glass bowl and set aside.
2. In a medium bowl, mix the hot water and coconut oil and let stand until the coconut oil melts.
3. Put the bentonite clay, stevia, and sea salt in the food processor and process until combined.
4. Add the water and coconut oil mixture gradually and process until combined.
5. With the machine running, add the essential oils and process for a few more seconds. The mixture should be granular and slightly damp.
6. Store in a glass jar with a lid.
7. Apply enough to cover your toothbrush. Wet with water and brush as normal.

Note: *To make the tooth powder into toothpaste, gradually add more coconut oil, blending as you go, until you reach the desired consistency.*

ESSENTIAL OIL–POWERED MOUTHWASH

10 drops essential oils (from the list of essential oil blends for oral care on page 148)

1 teaspoon carrier oil (not regular coconut oil, as it can harden and clog your pipes)

1 tablespoon alcohol-free witch hazel

1 teaspoon baking soda

1 cup distilled water

SUPPLIES

Mason jar for storage

1. In a mason jar, mix the essential oils with the carrier oil, witch hazel, baking soda, and filtered water and shake to blend.

2. When ready to use, swish approximately 1 tablespoon in the mouth for 10 to 15 seconds and rinse.

LICKABLE LIP BALM

For supple lips, lay this on thick and enjoy the flavor!

1 tablespoon beeswax

3 tablespoons organic, unrefined coconut oil

2½ teaspoons unrefined shea butter

5 drops vitamin E oil

3 drops ginger essential oil

2 drops peppermint essential oil

SUPPLIES

Small glass jar or measuring cup

Small saucepan

About 15 lip balm tubes or tins

1. Set a glass measuring cup or jar in a saucepan filled with an inch of water.
2. Place the beeswax, coconut oil, and shea butter in the jar and melt over medium heat, stirring occasionally.
3. When the ingredients are melted, remove the jar from the pan and quickly stir in the vitamin E and essential oils.
4. Carefully pour into tubes or small tins. Let cool.
5. Apply a small amount with your finger to ward off chapped lips.

Note: *If you are allergic to beeswax or are vegan, try candelilla wax or bayberry wax.*

ESSENTIAL OIL BLENDS FOR BEAUTY AND ANTI-AGING

- 20 drops helichrysum, 10 drops frankincense, 10 drops sandalwood, 5 drops lavender, 5 drops ylang ylang
- 20 drops ylang ylang, 10 drops geranium, 10 drops lavender, 10 drops rose absolute

ANTI-AGING BODY BUTTER

Look young and feel great with this soothing body butter.

1 cup unrefined shea butter
1 cup Mama Z's Oil Base (page 43)
50 drops essential oils (see the suggested blends above)

SUPPLIES
Small glass jar or measuring cup
Small saucepan
Medium glass bowl
Immersion blender or handheld mixer
Mason jar

1. Set a glass measuring cup or a jar in a saucepan filled with an inch of water.

2. Place the shea butter in the measuring cup or jar and melt over medium heat, stirring occasionally.

3. As soon as it's melted, remove measuring cup or jar from the pan and let cool.

4. Once it's cool enough to handle, pour the shea butter into a medium glass bowl.

5. Add Mama Z's Oil Base and the essential oils.

6. Chill in the refrigerator until partly solidified (about 15 minutes).

7. Whip to a butter-like consistency using an immersion blender or handheld mixer.

8. Store in a mason jar.

GARDENER'S HAND CREAM

From my Essential Oils Revolution cohost Jill Winger of ThePrairieHomestead .com: "Gardening can be hard on your hands, and this quick, homemade hand cream is perfect for dry or cracked skin. It's soothing and moisturizing, without being greasy."

¼ cup unrefined shea butter
1 tablespoon beeswax pastilles
2 tablespoons sweet almond oil
10 drops myrrh essential oil
10 drops cedarwood essential oil

SUPPLIES
Small glass jar
Small saucepan

1. Set a glass jar in a saucepan filled with an inch of water.

2. Place the shea butter, beeswax, and sweet almond oil in the jar and melt slowly over low heat, stirring occasionally.

3. Once everything is melted, remove the jar from the pan and allow it to cool for 5 to 10 minutes.

4. Stir in the essential oils. Allow it to harden completely (this usually takes several hours, but refrigerating can speed up the process).

5. Apply this cream to your dry hands as often as needed—especially after a long day working outside or playing in the dirt.

Note: *If you are allergic to beeswax or are vegan, try candelilla wax or bayberry wax.*

DEET-FREE BUG SPRAY

This all-natural insect repellent made with pure essential oils is safe for the whole family.

1 ounce carrier oil of choice
3 drops citronella essential oil
3 drops eucalyptus essential oil
3 drops tea tree essential oil
3 drops peppermint essential oil
3 drops cypress essential oil
3 drops lemon myrtle essential oil

SUPPLIES
1-ounce spray bottle

1. Mix all the ingredients in a small glass spray bottle and store in a cool dark place.

2. Spritz over the entire body before heading outside, being careful to avoid your eyes as essential oils are strong and will burn.

3. Reapply every couple of hours you're outside.

SOOTHING BUG BITE BALM

5 drops peppermint essential oil
5 drops lavender essential oil
Fractionated coconut oil as needed

SUPPLIES
5 ml glass roller bottle

1. Drop the essential oils into the roller bottle.
2. Fill the bottle with fractionated coconut oil and shake well.
3. Apply to bug bites as needed to relieve itch and sting.

STINK NO MORE DEODORANT

2 to 4 tablespoons organic coconut oil
2 tablespoons cocoa butter
2 tablespoons unrefined shea butter
¼ cup arrowroot powder
1 tablespoon baking soda
1½ teaspoons non-GMO organic cornstarch
15 drops essential oils

SUPPLIES
1-pint mason or other glass jar
Small saucepan
1 empty stick deodorant container

1. Set a jar in a saucepan filled with an inch of water.
2. Place 2 tablespoons of the coconut oil, the cocoa butter, and shea butter in the jar and melt slowly over low heat, stirring occasionally.
3. As soon as you are able to stir the mixture, remove the jar from the heat so it's not too hot for the other ingredients.
4. Stir in the arrowroot, baking soda, and cornstarch.
5. Stir in the essential oils.

6. When the mixture is still pourable but thick enough to not be runny, fill the empty stick deodorant container. (Make sure the applicator is rolled all the way down so there is room for the mixture!)

7. Store in a cool, dry place and apply as you would regular stick deodorant.

Note: *Some of my favorite essential oils for a deodorant are cedarwood, clary sage, geranium, lemon, lavender, tea tree, jasmine absolute, lemongrass, sweet or wild orange, rose absolute, sandalwood, ylang ylang, and vanilla absolute.*

Don't forget that certain citrus oils are photosensitizing, so be sure not to apply a citrus-based deodorant before sunbathing or when your underarms will be at risk of burning due to sun exposure.

Also, if your mixture starts melting in the summer, try adding 1 to 2 tablespoons of kokum butter, which is the hardest butter available (you can purchase it online from many different retailers, including Amazon). You will need to add 4 or 5 more drops of essential oils to overcome the waxy smell of the kokum butter.

A Special Note About Acne

Since various bacteria can cause skin breakouts, treating acne can be tricky. One thing we do know, however, is that antibiotics are often not the answer because antimicrobial resistance has developed in bacterial strains involved in the development of acne. Thus, researchers are looking for viable natural solutions, and essential oils keep proving themselves to be effective acne remedies.[6]

In one time-tested study evaluating how ten different essential oils killed *Propionibacterium acnes*, thyme, cinnamon bark, and rose were the three most effective at killing the acne-causing bacteria completely within five minutes.[7] Before you start slathering yourself with thyme and cinnamon bark, remember that these oils have a tendency to irritate the skin. Be sure to work with your skin type, dilute properly, and use a gentler blend if necessary.

Another evaluation created a gel formulation based on orange (*Citrus sinensis*) and sweet basil (*Ocimum basilicum* L).[8] Of the twenty-eight people who participated in this particular study, every single one reported an improvement ranging between 43 percent and 75 percent clearance of their blemishes. The researchers found that this particular formulation was so gentle on the skin, little discomfort and few side effects were reported.

ACNE TREATMENT ROLL-ON

1 drop cinnamon bark essential oil

1 drop rose essential oil

2 drops thyme essential oil

Fractionated coconut oil (this carrier works best because it doesn't leave an oily residue on your skin)

SUPPLIES

10 ml glass roller bottle

1. Drop the essential oils into the roller bottle.
2. Fill the roller bottle with fractionated coconut oil.
3. Spot-treat blemishes after washing your face in the morning and at night.

Note: *Discontinue use immediately if burning or irritation occurs, and consider trying a more soothing gel for sensitive skin (recipe follows).*

ACNE TREATMENT SOOTHING GEL FOR SENSITIVE SKIN

3 drops sweet or wild orange essential oil

3 drops basil essential oil

1 teaspoon aloe vera gel

Fractionated coconut oil

SUPPLIES

1-ounce glass pump dispenser

1. Drop the essential oils into the pump dispenser.
2. Add the aloe and shake gently.
3. Fill the bottle with fractionated coconut oil and shake gently to mix.
4. Spot-treat blemishes after washing your face in the morning and at night.

10

Around the House

Homes should be an anchor, a safe harbor, a place of refuge, a place where families dwell together, a place where children are loved.

—L. TOM PERRY

You may have the most lovingly decorated and cared-for home that instantly puts you, your family, and anyone who comes to visit you at ease. But no matter how nurturing your surroundings, if you're using conventional cleaning products with heavy fragrances and scented candles and air fresheners, you're creating a toxic environment that can be putting your health in jeopardy.

This is what happened to Shawn and Natalie, a young couple with three kids who were seeking an answer to why their kids were always succumbing to viruses and why the whole family was experiencing worse and worse seasonal allergies each year. That's how they stumbled on my website and signed up for an upcoming online health summit, where I shared the two things I suggest everyone do to improve their health:

1. First, throw away hand sanitizers and antibacterial products, and start to DIY (because of all the reasons shared in chapter 9).
2. Second, toss all your air fresheners in the can and use essential oils instead because the chemicals in fake scents are known carcinogens and neurotoxins.

Inspired by my talk, Shawn and Natalie stopped using their expensive plug-in air fresheners and threw their bathroom aerosols in the trash. Once they were using only essential oils spritzers and diffusers to enhance the smell of their home, their allergies all but disappeared.

THE DANGERS LURKING IN ARTIFICIAL FRAGRANCES

Similar to how antibacterial agents like triclosan are now public health enemy number one in the body care industry, artificial fragrances hold that title in the household cleaning industry. Due to what's referred to as the "fragrance loophole," federal law does not mandate that the ingredients making up these synthetic aromas be listed individually.

Labels sport the generic term *fragrance* or *parfum*, and millions of unsuspecting consumers are duped into inhaling mini-doses of chemicals like styrene, a known human carcinogen, when they use scented home and body care items.[1] These chemicals are linked to a variety of conditions ranging from asthma to neurotoxicity, and their presence seems almost inescapable.[2]

Thankfully, we have a choice in the products that we buy. Products that are made from natural ingredients eliminate many of the chemicals that are present in artificial scents. Many essential oils offer fresh and amazing scents, and they have none of the three thousand chemicals that make up these toxic aromas.[3]

The next logical step is to start cutting down on the number of scented products you use. Do you really need scented dryer sheets? Can you replace commercial cleaners with those you can make at home? Be a little more willing to read labels and a little braver about trying natural products.

Similar to its Skin Deep Cosmetics Database, the EWG has created a database that ranks more than 2,500 store-bought cleaners according to safety. Check out where your favorites rank at http://www.EWG.org/Guides/Cleaners.

ALL-NATURAL, SWEET-SMELLING CLEANING PRODUCTS

Replacing toxic air fresheners is supereasy in the aromatherapy world. Just use your diffuser! (For a list of essential oils that are good air purifiers, refer to the list of top note essential oils in the Aromatic Note Classification list on page 49.)

Replacing other products is not as quick, but it's certainly doable, and very cost-effective. The first step is to toss all those chemicals in the trash; then start to make your own. Below you'll find recipes for all of the products you need to get started.

Remember, typical household cleansers are loaded with toxic chemicals—they may produce the clean results you're looking for, but those chemicals remain in the air and on the surfaces you touch every day, contributing to indoor air pollution. While there are many better, "natural" cleaning products on the market, these make-your-own versions work every bit as well, smell great, and are much less expensive!

LEMON FRESH LAUNDRY DETERGENT

This recipe will wash up to 150 loads for less than $20.

½ bar Dr. Bronner's unscented castile soap
5 cups distilled water
¾ cup OxiClean Baby Stain Remover
¾ cup Arm & Hammer Super Washing Soda Household Cleaner & Laundry Booster
One 5 ml bottle of any essential oil (lemongrass, lavender, and ylang ylang all work great; a basic guideline to how many drops is 100 per 5 ml bottle)

SUPPLIES
Large stockpot
Three 1-gallon glass jars with pump dispensers (available on Amazon) (5-gallon heavy-duty plastic buckets with a lid for storage work as well)

1. Grate the entire bar of soap into the stockpot over low heat.
2. Add the water and raise the heat to medium-high. Stir until the soap is dissolved.

3. Add the OxiClean and washing soda and mix until dissolved.

4. Remove from the heat and let cool for a few minutes.

5. Pour 1 quart hot water into each of the three containers.

6. Add 2 cups of the soap mixture and 30 drops of essential oil into each container. Stir, then add enough cool water to fill each container.

7. Let the mixture thicken overnight. (If using a plastic bucket, use the lid.)

8. Depending on whether you have a high-efficiency washer, use between ¼ and ½ cup per load.

Notes: *Stir (if using a plastic bucket for storage) or shake (if storing in a glass bottle) before each use as the detergent may get lumpy or gelatinous.*

Also, in case you were wondering, the nonprofit watchdog Environmental Working Group gives both Arm & Hammer Super Washing Soda and OxiClean Baby Stain Remover an "A" grade because they have virtually no associated toxic risks. The known ingredients are sodium carbonate peroxide and sodium carbonate, which are both very safe and effective at removing stains.

TEA TREE CITRUS BATHROOM CLEANER

The star of this blend is orange essential oil, which is a known mood booster. You'll be happier even though you're stuck cleaning the bathroom!

2 tablespoons Dr. Bronner's liquid castile soap
2 tablespoons baking soda
20 drops tea tree essential oil
15 drops orange or lemon essential oil (or 7 drops of each)
15 drops lemon eucalyptus or lemon myrtle essential oil
2 cups distilled water

SUPPLIES
32-ounce spray bottle, preferably glass

1. Combine the liquid soap, baking soda, and essential oils in the spray bottle and mix well.

2. Pour in the water and shake well.

3. Use as you would any other bathroom cleaner. Shake before each use.

JUNIPER TOILET DEODORIZING SPRAY

Freshen up your toilet with this woodsy, clean scent!

1 ounce witch hazel

10 drops vitamin E (as a preservative)

20 drops juniper berry essential oil

20 drops cypress essential oil

10 drops pine essential oil

Distilled water

SUPPLIES

2-ounce spray bottle, preferably glass

1. Combine the witch hazel, vitamin E, and essential oils in the bottle and mix well.

2. Pour in enough distilled water to fill the bottle and shake well.

3. Spray twice into the toilet as needed for a fresh smell.

OTHER BATHROOM-CLEANING BLENDS

Use 25 drops essential oil per 1 ounce of liquid.

- Key lime, opoponax, and vanilla absolute
- Geranium, lavender, rose absolute, and ylang ylang
- Lemon, lemon tea tree, lemongrass, and tea tree

CITRUS ABRASIVE CLEANSER

This formula is great for cleaning sinks, pans, stovetops, and more.

½ cup baking soda
5 drops lemon essential oil
5 drops sweet or wild orange essential oil
5 drops grapefruit essential oil

SUPPLIES
Glass shaker jar

1. Combine the baking soda and essential oils in a glass jar and shake until thoroughly mixed. The mixture will be powdery.
2. Use as you would a normal cleanser—sprinkle a bit on the surface you want to clean, then use a damp cloth to make a bit of a paste and scrub. Wipe away with a clean damp cloth.

Notes: *I like cheese shakers for this because they make it easy to use, but any glass jar will do.*

For a little extra cleaning power, spray the soiled area with white vinegar before sprinkling on the cleanser and add an extra drop of one of the essential oils to the surface.

PICK-YOUR-OIL TILE CLEANER

Mix and match the essential oils to fit your needs—and watch this cleaner kill everything from mold to dust mites!

1 gallon hot distilled water
¼ cup vinegar
2 tablespoons Dr. Bronner's liquid castile soap
20 drops essential oils (see the list below)

SUPPLIES
Mop bucket

1. Fill a mop bucket with hot water first to prevent a soap bubble overflow.
2. Add the vinegar, soap, and essential oils and stir well.
3. Use this cleanser to mop your tile floor or clean your bathtub.
4. Store any leftovers in a large unbreakable bottle or bucket with a lid.

ESSENTIAL OILS FOR CLEANING GLASS

- Bergamot
- Grapefruit
- Lemon
- Lime
- Neroli
- Tangerine
- Wild orange

CITRUS-POWERED GLASS CLEANER

Any and all citrus oils work—find your favorite blend!

½ teaspoon Dr. Bronner's liquid castile soap
¼ cup white vinegar
25 drops citrus essential oils (see the list above)
Distilled water, as needed

SUPPLIES
16-ounce glass spray bottle

1. Pour the soap, vinegar, and essential oils into the spray bottle.
2. Fill the rest of the bottle with distilled water, screw on the pump, and shake heavily.
3. Spray directly on glass windows and mirrors for cleaning.

ESSENTIAL OILS FOR TOUGH CLEANING JOBS

- Citronella wards off bugs.
- Eucalyptus kills dust mites.
- Lemon kills bacteria.
- Pine and fir needle are antiseptic and leave a pleasant smell.
- Tea tree is an antifungal and kills mold.

LEMON TEA TREE DISH SOAP

½ cup Dr. Bronner's liquid castile soap

2 teaspoons vegetable glycerin (available at many household goods stores and online at Amazon.com)

6 drops lemon essential oil

4 drops tea tree essential oil

4 drops lemon eucalyptus or lemon myrtle essential oil (or 2 drops each)

Distilled water as needed

SUPPLIES

16-ounce glass bottle with pump or glass foaming soap dispenser

1. Pour the liquid castile soap and vegetable glycerin into the glass bottle.
2. Add the essential oils.
3. Fill the bottle with distilled water, allowing room for the pump. Replace the pump.
4. Shake well and use like you would traditional dish soap.

→ To watch me and Mama Z make this dish soap recipe and show you how we organize our kitchen cleaning products, go to HealingPowerOfEssentialOils.com.

KITCHEN COUNTER SPRAY

Streak-free, fresh-smelling counters are just a few ingredients away!

4 ounces white vinegar (see Note)
10 drops lemongrass essential oil
10 drops tea tree essential oil
5 drops lemon eucalyptus essential oil
5 drops citronella essential oil
1 cup distilled water

SUPPLIES
16-ounce glass spray bottle

1. Pour all the ingredients into a glass spray bottle and shake to evenly combine.
2. Spray your kitchen counters and wipe down.

Note: *Vinegar can damage granite counter tops. Replace the vinegar with 70% isopropyl alcohol or vodka.*

CITRUS DUSTING SPRAY

The dust in your home doesn't stand a chance with this citrus-powered spray.

4 ounces carrier oil
5 drops lemon myrtle essential oil
5 drops lemon eucalyptus oil
5 drops tangerine essential oil

SUPPLIES
4-ounce glass spray bottle with a mister attachment

1. Combine all the ingredients in a spray bottle.
2. Spray liberally on all your wood surfaces. Wipe off with a soft, clean cloth.

GARDEN PEST SPRAY

When you're growing an organic garden, pests can be a real problem. Use this simple formulation to save your veggies from hungry insects and other critters—no chemicals required. You'll see just how effective essential oils can be in your outdoor spaces! Just be sure to wash any produce thoroughly after harvesting before you eat it.

20 drops peppermint essential oil
20 drops rosemary essential oil
20 drops clove essential oil
¼ teaspoon natural liquid dish soap
Distilled water, as needed

SUPPLIES
1-quart spray bottle

1. Combine the essential oils and dish soap in a spray bottle. Fill the rest of the bottle with distilled water, and gently shake to combine.
2. Spray on the leaves of plants being targeted by pests.
3. Repeat frequently, especially after rain or watering.

Note: *Always do a test on a small portion of the plant before spraying your entire crop. I've never had the spray cause an adverse reaction, but it's better to be safe than sorry. Also, avoid spraying during the heat of the day.*

11

Essential Oils for Athletes

My grandmother started walking five miles a day when she was sixty. She's ninety-seven now, and we don't know where the heck she is.

—*ELLEN DEGENERES*

ssential oils can help athletes of all ages in a plethora of ways, and in this chapter I share some effective DIY recipes clinically proven to enhance energy and soothe achy muscles. I even give practical tips to combat stinky gear naturally. But first, it's superimportant that we quickly discuss one of the most widely used (and abused) tools in the average athlete's tool belt: energy drinks.

This is a must-read for all athletes, especially the recipes and tips that show you how to use essential oils to naturally boost energy levels!

TOO MUCH CAFFEINE: THE HEALTH RISKS ASSOCIATED WITH ENERGY DRINKS

Despite the thirty-year energy drink craze that has now become a vast $50 billion-plus global market, I plead with everyone consuming these products to stop immediately![1] As one study bluntly puts it, "Energy drinks have no therapeutic benefit, and many ingredients are understudied and not regulated. The known and unknown pharmacology of agents included in such drinks, combined with reports of toxicity, raises concern for potentially serious adverse effects in association with energy drink use."[2]

What's the big deal, you may be asking? Well, for starters, each energy drink contains the caffeine of up to five cups of coffee. Just think about that for a moment. Five cups! When people chug two, three, or even four energy drinks, they consume more caffeine in one day than a one-cup-per-day coffee drinker does in two weeks!

I cannot even begin to stress how dangerous energy drinks are for you. Studies have shown that the excessive caffeine in these power drinks may cause vomiting, cardiac arrhythmias, seizures, and even death.[3] These symptoms have all been reported as known concerns by the National Center for Complementary and Integrative Health.[4]

As a public health initiative, it's important to note that, despite knowing that nearly 50 percent of college athletes use various energy drinks, we do not yet have the data to tell us how many postcollege athletes use them.[5] The studies simply have not been done. Still, casual observance has led me to conclude that many older adult athletes use them because I have seen a stark increase among people at fitness centers and local sporting events drinking caffeinated performance boosters. If you're anything like me, you see people with energy drinks all over the place—everywhere from church softball games to bowling alleys to golf outings. This should not surprise us, as sales of caffeinated energy drinks and shots have experienced double-digit growth in the past few years.[6]

Misuse of caffeinated energy drinks has actually become a global epidemic. A fantastic review published in the *Drug and Alcohol Dependence* journal states: "Hundreds of different brands are now marketed, with caffeine content ranging from a modest 50 mg to an alarming 505 mg per can or bottle. Regulation of energy drinks, including content labeling and health warnings, differs across countries, with some of the most lax regulatory requirements in the U.S."[7]

Don't get me wrong, I enjoy the caffeine rush that I get in my matcha green tea latte and occasional cup of organic coffee, but it's important to set some limits. Up to 505 milligrams of caffeine per bottle is ridiculous to consume in one sitting. For comparison, that's equivalent to four to five cups of coffee in one can![8] The problem is that, unlike slowly drinking five cups of coffee over several hours or even days, people down these energy drinks like shots at the bar. Many of them are actually sold as shots!

The question begging to be asked at this point is, "Can essential oils replace caffeine?"

Yes, I believe they can, and I'll show you how!

SUGAR: THE REAL INGREDIENT THAT GIVES PEOPLE A "BOOST"

It has long been documented that Red Bull improves physical and cognitive performance.[9] However, something interesting happens when sugar is taken out of the mix. According to multiple double-blind placebo trials testing *sugar-free* Red Bull, these versions of the drink do not enhance performance. In testing the time-to-exhaustion for high-intensity runs and blood lactate levels (two indicators assessing exercise capacity), as well as perceived levels of exertion, sugar-free energy drinks failed to help at all.[10] Studies have also shown that sugar-free energy drinks have no effect on upper body strength and muscular endurance.[11]

As research suggests, sugar-free energy drinks are not effective at doing much besides creating intense caffeine intoxication, addiction, and withdrawal.[12] Since sugar is the only missing ingredient in sugar-free Red Bull, logic leads us to conclude that the caffeine and taurine aren't doing the trick.

Obviously, it's the sugar that's making the big difference, which make sense because long-distance, high-intensity athletes of all ages fall prey to the marketing ploys of manufacturers that sell sugar-filled bars, gels, jelly beans, and sports drinks. Thus, not counting the obvious danger in consuming too much caffeine, the extreme amounts of sugar that many energy drinks contain (up to 50 grams, or 10 teaspoons, per 8-ounce serving!) puts people at risk of developing diabetes, obesity, and other sugar-related illnesses.

THE DANGER OF TOO MUCH TAURINE

These performance boosters also contain excessive amounts of other ingredients like taurine, a supplementary amino acid in Red Bull (1,000 mg), Monster (2,000 mg), and Rockstar (3,000 mg).[13] In its natural form, taurine is cardioprotective, and up to 3,000 milligrams a day is generally considered safe.[14] Moderation is important because little is known about the effects of heavy or long-term taurine use, and there is a legitimate concern that people who regularly drink two, three, or more energy drinks per day can easily exceed the maximum daily limit recognized by the Food and Drug Administration.[15] At one point, Norway, Denmark, and France had banned the sale of Red Bull, partly in response to a study on rats that were fed taurine and exhibited bizarre behavior, including anxiety and self-mutilation.[16] Interestingly, there is little to no evidence of the impact of high doses of taurine on physical activity, whereas studies have shown that moderate doses of 500 milligrams three times per day can increase exercise time and distance effectively in older patients (with a mean age of 60) with heart failure.[17]

A SPECIAL NOTE TO CAREGIVERS

I know many of you reading this book are parents, grandparents, teachers, and caregivers, so please be aware that children are in danger of developing serious health issues from consuming energy drinks. In fact, a study published in the journal *Current Opinion in Pediatrics* stresses the growing concern that teenagers who regularly consume Red Bull, Monster, and other so-called performance enhancers are particularly at risk of developing serious health concerns:[18]

- Disrupted sleep patterns
- Elevated blood pressure
- Exacerbated psychiatric disease
- Increased risk of subsequent addiction (a gateway drug)
- Physiologic dependence

Please keep this in mind if you see the young adults in your life drinking these dangerous energy boosters. Often all it takes is just one caring word from a teacher, parent, or another loved one to steer them in the right direction. (And if that falls on deaf ears, scare them straight with a dose of science!)

HOW TO USE ESSENTIAL OILS FOR IMPROVED WORKOUTS, FASTER RECOVERY, AND BETTER-SMELLING GEAR

Essential oils can be powerful, useful tools for athletes. No matter your expertise or skill level, there is a natural solution for you. Here are just four of the many reasons every athlete should use essential oils.

1. Performance Boosters

Ingesting peppermint in water has been tested extensively for its performance-boosting abilities. Controlled experiments with athletes have demonstrated *instant* improvement in performance measures like jumping, grip strength, endurance, and respiration.[19] Peppermint improves bronchial smooth-muscle tonicity, which helps people breathe better by expanding their lung capacity. As an extra bonus, increased oxygen delivery helps your cells burn fat more efficiently!

According to multiple studies out of Iran, ingesting peppermint oil affects blood pressure, breathing, and other physiological measures.[20] Additionally, topical application and inhalation have been shown to improve pain tolerance and workload capacity.[21] Add peppermint to your training regimen—whether internally, topically, or inhaled—to boost your athletic performance ability in a proven, natural way.

Safety Note: In spite of the research suggesting that mixing peppermint oil into a glass of water can enhance athletic performance, this practice is not a long-term solution. A better way to ingest peppermint essential oil is to put 1 or 2 drops in a gel capsule filled with an edible carrier oil. Alternatively, you can mix 1 or 2 drops of peppermint with a teaspoon of coconut oil and consume. Here's why: Peppermint is such a profound muscle relaxer, that consuming undiluted peppermint oil has the tendency to cause acid reflux because it can prevent the esophageal sphincter from closing properly. Your esophageal sphincter performs like a valve, preventing contents from your gastric cavity from rising up into your esophagus. When this valve isn't functioning properly, acid from your stomach rises up and causes heartburn.

Applications:

- Consume 1 drop of peppermint oil with 1 teaspoon of organic, unrefined coconut oil right before your workout. Coconut oil has also been shown to enhance athletic endurance, so this is a one-two punch of natural energy.[22]
- Alternatively, you can consume 2 drops of peppermint oil in a size 00 gel capsule filled with coconut oil to prevent the oil from coming into contact with your oral cavity and esophagus.
- Apply a 2%–3% dilution of peppermint oil mixed with unrefined coconut oil over your chest and the back of your neck for a pre- and post-workout pick-me-up. The VOCs will jump off your skin and keep you energized throughout your entire workout.
- Make my Performance Booster Inhaler.

Safety Tip: Be careful when taking peppermint straight with your water. Similar to how it relaxes your bronchial smooth muscles, it can relax your esophageal sphincter and cause reflux.

PERFORMANCE BOOSTER INHALER

10 drops peppermint essential oil
5 drops sweet or wild orange essential oil
5 drops spearmint essential oil

SUPPLIES
Precut organic cotton pad
Aromatherapy inhaler

1. Place a cotton pad in the inhaler tube.
2. Drop the essential oils directly onto the cotton pad inside the tube. Alternatively, you can drop the essential oils into a glass bowl, roll the cotton pad in the oils to absorb them, and then insert it into the inhaler tube using tweezers.

3. Open the inhaler and take five deep breaths before your workout or between sets.

4. Keep on hand for those long runs and extended workouts!

➡ To watch me and Mama Z make this Performance Booster Inhaler and learn how we like to stay energized during our workouts, go to HealingPowerOfEssentialOils.com.

2. Relief for Achy Muscles

You may have your fair share of aches, pains, and sore muscles after an intense training session. Two oils that have been shown to help with pain are lavender and peppermint (which happen to pair quite well!).

Lavender

The mainstay of essential oils, lavender was studied in 2014 for its effects on neck pain. The oil was added to a cream that participants massaged onto the painful area daily. The essential oil cream was more effective at reducing pain levels than the non-EO control.[23]

Peppermint

As noted earlier, peppermint can help minimize pain that's been triggered by athletic pursuits. It's well known for its analgesic properties, as well as its antispasmodic properties for those with tight muscles.[24] The cooling sensation of peppermint as well as the uplifting scent also make it perfect for reviving yourself after a hard day of training.

Traditional Oils

Many oils, such as fir oil, have traditionally been used for pain relief. Ayurvedic practices cite the use of fir essential oil as the "forest healer" for various kinds of joint and muscle pain relief.[25] Wintergreen, marjoram, and frankincense are also known for deep pain relief and work wonderfully together.

Application: Try my Extra-Strength Muscle-Soothing Body Oil, designed just for hard-working athletes!

EXTRA-STRENGTH MUSCLE-SOOTHING BODY OIL

Note that this is a strong 5% dilution recipe. If you experience any sort of irritation, add more carrier oil for a dilution suited to your skin type.

50 drops frankincense essential oil
50 drops peppermint essential oil
20 drops sweet marjoram essential oil
20 drops lavender essential oil
10 drops wintergreen essential oil
5 ounces Mama Z's Oil Base (page 43)

SUPPLIES
Medium glass bowl
6-ounce glass lotion dispenser or glass salve jar

1. Drop the essential oils into a medium glass bowl.
2. Add Mama Z's base and mix.
3. Rub over sore muscles after workouts or on off days.
4. Store in a lotion dispenser or glass jar in the refrigerator.

3. Antimicrobial Healing

Sometimes it's scrapes and cuts that need a remedy, not just aches and pains. A rough slide into home plate, a fall on the track—athletic ventures put your body through the wringer, and sometimes across the pavement!

Instead of over-the-counter antibiotic ointments, make a simple DIY injury spray with astringent witch hazel and antimicrobial essential oils. Keep it in your gym or equipment bag just in case.

Application: Use the hand sanitizer recipe from chapter 9 (page 144) as a base and make a blend of special wound-healing essential oils from proven oils like basil, frankincense, geranium, lavender, myrrh, Roman chamomile, and tea tree in a ratio of 15 drops of essential oil per ounce.

4. Nontoxic Solution to Stinky Sports Gear

Freshen up that smelly athletic gear with antimicrobial and lemon-scented essential oils. Start off by making a special blend that I originally created to combat a musty basement odor.

LEMON FRESH BLEND

For a 5 ml bottle, you need:

40 drops: Lemon essential oil
20 drops: Lemon basil essential oil
20 drops: Lemon eucalyptus essential oil
20 drops: Lemon myrtle essential oil
20 drops: Lemon tea tree essential oil

Add 5 or 6 drops of this recipe to a portable car or USB diffuser after a game or in your gym bag or gear storage area to freshen things up a bit. It's also great in my Odor-Eating Powder and Stinky Gear Spray recipes (page 176).

Note: *For a different quantity, simply remember that you want two parts lemon essential oil to one part of each of the other oils.*

ODOR-EATING POWDER

20 drops Lemon Fresh Blend (page 175)
½ cup baking soda

SUPPLIES
Glass shaker jar

1. Combine the ingredients in the jar and shake well to distribute.
2. Before a workout or game, sprinkle the powder inside your shoes or on top of stinky gear.
3. For extra odor protection, apply after a workout or game when you put away your shoes for the night.
4. Store the mixture in the fridge—it should last for a few weeks.

Notes: *Alternatively, you can use the following Stinky Gear Spray.*

You can also shake some of this blend on your carpet—then vacuum to freshen up the house!

STINKY GEAR SPRAY

5 ml Lemon Fresh Blend (page 175)
2 ounces apple cider vinegar
2 ounces witch hazel
4 ounces distilled water

SUPPLIES
8-ounce glass spray bottle

1. Pour the essential oils, vinegar, and witch hazel into the spray bottle.
2. Mix by swirling together.
3. Add the water and shake vigorously.
4. Spritz over your gear after a workout or when needed.

12

Using Essential Oils with Your Animals

The greatness of a nation can be judged by the way its animals are treated.

—MAHATMA GANDHI

specialize in public health and essential oils research for people, not animals. Yet, in spite of not knowing the first thing about animals, I have some friends who do.

Since I get asked about how to use essential oils with animals quite regularly, I made sure that I interviewed animal aromatherapy experts during both my Essential Oils Revolution 1 and 2 summits. Based on my collaboration with animal aromatherapist and veterinarian Janet Roark, this chapter is a collection of the key takeaways that I have gleaned from the interviews and articles that we've worked on together. To follow Dr. Roark's work, find her on Facebook at Essential Oil Vet— Janet Roark, DVM (@EODVM).

→ To listen to one of my special interviews with Dr. Roark, go to HealingPowerOfEssentialOils.com.

ANIMAL AROMATHERAPY BASICS

It is somewhat ironic that many pet owners will place toxic air fresheners in every room throughout their house without thinking twice, but wonder if diffusing essential oils will harm their pets! Putting things into perspective is key.

As a rule of thumb, you want to approach using essential oils with your pets like you would with babies and small children. Although they cannot speak, your animals each have their own preferences and sensitivities, so it is important to observe your pets' behavior. If your animal is behaving normally, all is well. If he is behaving abnormally, then he may be sensitive to an oil you are using. Pets are very good at telling you what they need.

By following Dr. Roark's advice below, you'll be able to start using essential oils safely on and around your pets.

Large Animals

With full-grown large animal herbivores, such as alpacas, cattle, horses, llamas, sheep, and goats, you can apply essential oils topically on an area of concern as you would apply them to a human. Note that newborn and young large animals require greater dilution.

Small Animals

With small animals such as cats and dogs, you will need to dilute more heavily. Use these specific guidelines for your small pets:

Birds

Birds are very sensitive to essential oils, so water diffusion is advised in lieu of topical application. Lavender and citrus oils are great mood enhancers. Be sure to avoid "hot" oils like lemongrass, clove, and cinnamon bark or cinnamon leaf, which are frequently in many immunity support blends on the market. Also, be careful to diffuse your oils in a well-ventilated room. Just as with babies, you don't want to shut your bird in a small room with a diffuser running all night!

Cats

Because cats lack an enzyme in their liver that helps metabolize many chemicals, they are susceptible to toxicity from a wide variety of sources, including poisonous plants, nonsteroidal anti-inflammatory medications (like aspirin and ibuprofen), acetaminophen, chocolate, caffeine, methylxanthines, lead, zinc, and many types of pesticides. Also be sure to avoid oils high in ketones and phenols (two substances that are metabolized by the liver) when applying oils topically or internally, including:

Basil	Oregano
Birch	Peppermint
Cinnamon bark or cinnamon	Tea tree
leaf	Thyme
Clove	Rosemary
Fennel	Spearmint
Nutmeg	Wintergreen

Cats are also sensitive to oils containing d-limonene, so avoid these as well:

Bergamot	Lime
Dill	Orange
Grapefruit	Tangerine
Lemon	

Dogs

In general, the smaller the dog, the more you want to dilute essential oils. There is some concern in the aromatherapy community about using certain oils on dogs, such as birch, camphor, tea tree, and wintergreen, so it would be wise to avoid using them directly on your dogs because there are so many alternatives that aren't controversial.

Pocket Pets

Chinchillas, guinea pigs, hamsters, rabbits, and sugar gliders rely on friendly bacteria to help digest their food, so you want to be very careful when using essential oils with strong antibacterial properties, such as cinnamon bark, cinnamon leaf, thyme, tea tree, and oregano. Since these animals have delicate digestive flora, you do not want to inadvertently disrupt them by using essential oils.

CONSIDERATIONS WHEN WORKING WITH ANIMALS WITH SPECIAL NEEDS

- **Bleeding disorders.** For those animals that have difficulty clotting or are being treated with an anticoagulant, be sure to avoid topical application of birch, cassia, cinnamon bark, cinnamon leaf, clove, fennel, oregano, and wintergreen.
- **Seizure disorders.** Some oils are thought to lower the seizure threshold, so be sure to avoid those oils. They include basil, black pepper, camphor, eucalyptus, fennel, hyssop, sage, rosemary, and wintergreen.
- **Pregnant or nursing animals.** All essential oils should be highly diluted. Oils to avoid include basil, cassia, cinnamon bark, cinnamon leaf, clary sage, rosemary, thyme, wintergreen, and white fir.

ESSENTIAL OIL REMEDIES FOR COMMON ANIMAL AILMENTS

- **Allergies.** This is a somewhat complex topic to generalize for all pets, but with dogs and large animals, it is advisable to (carefully) give frankincense, lemon, lavender, and peppermint two or three times daily with animals on their feet in addition to omega-3 supplementation. It's always a good idea to work with your veterinarian in these cases to determine the source of the allergy, because addressing the root cause will help prevent itching. Sometimes it takes a while to figure it out, but it is well worth it!
- **Fear-based issues.** For behavioral issues such as separation anxiety, thunderstorm anxiety, and fear or fear-based aggression, you can diffuse calming oils throughout the house and apply a 0.5%–1% dilution of lavender alone or a combination of lavender and vetiver over their fur with great success. Just be sure not to apply it on any areas where your pet can reach to lick it off. The DIY anti-anxiety spray recipe I include on page 181 can also help.
- **Ear infections.** Cleaning your pets' ears regularly with a natural ear cleaner is essential. After cleaning, apply a 0.5%–1% blend of basil, frankincense, geranium, and lavender around the base of the ear for added support.

- **Neoplasia.** Uncomplicated cases of abnormal tissue growth can benefit from 0.5%–1% diluted topical support with frankincense and sandalwood. I always recommend consulting with a veterinary oncologist in these cases.
- **Seizures.** Adding 1 or 2 drops of frankincense to food twice daily as well as omega-3 supplementation can help considerably.
- **Transitions.** Diffusing calming oils and applying a 0.5%–1% blend of lavender and myrrh can really help with an adjustment period such as bringing a new puppy home, transitioning between homes, or adding a new animal to a herd.
- **Lyme disease.** Protecting your pet from fleas and ticks will also protect you and your family from their bites—and the potential of getting Lyme disease, which is a threat to both the two-legged and four-legged members of your family! Store the simple, fabulous-smelling spray on page 182 in a glass bottle, then spritz on their fur before you head out. (It will also help ward off any musty pet smells on your furniture and rugs, as it doubles as an odor eliminator.)

ANTI-ANXIETY SPRAY

This spray is a powerful DIY tool to calm your pet's nerves.

1 drop lavender essential oil
1 drop frankincense essential oil
1 drop vetiver essential oil
Distilled water, as needed

SUPPLIES
2-ounce glass spray bottle

1. Combine the oils in the spray bottle and fill with distilled water.
2. Shake well before each use.
3. Mist your animal's back and bedding, and/or diffuse in the home while you are away.

ANXIETY DOG COLLAR

Premix a frankincense, lavender, and vetiver blend (with a carrier oil, of course, in a 1% dilution) and apply 2 drops directly on the back of your animal's collar or bridle.

FLEA AND TICK REPELLENT

Although these essential oils are generally safe for dogs and cats, remember that pets have allergies just like humans do, so keep a close eye on them to make sure they do not have a negative reaction. Also, be careful not to spray around your pet's face.

2 tablespoons sweet almond oil
1 drop lavender essential oil
1 drop grapefruit essential oil
1 drop eucalyptus essential oil
1 drop lemongrass essential oil

SUPPLIES
8-ounce glass spray bottle

1. Combine the almond oil and essential oils in the bottle.
2. Fill the rest of the bottle with water and shake to mix.
3. Spray on your pet's coat before heading outside, taking care to avoid the face.
4. Shake well before each use.

BEHAVIORS TO WATCH FOR

Since every animal is different and has a unique body chemistry, pets' tolerance of essential oils will vary. For example, Dr. Roark's puppy loves a wide variety of essential oils and can handle most applications, but her older Scottish terrier is much more sensitive and prefers diffusion only.

As I mentioned above, it's important to simply observe your pet's behavior. If she's behaving normally, all is well. If she's behaving abnormally, such as trying to rub the oil off her fur, squinting, rubbing her nose, or trying to get out of a room where you are diffusing, then your pet may be sensitive to a particular oil or blend.

For the most part, your animals will experience the same therapeutic effect that humans enjoy. Remember, most research studies and product testing are done on animals! While I am not providing an entire chapter's worth of recipes specific to your pets, the good news is that you can whip up many of the same recipes that are designed for humans and just slightly tweak how you use them with your furry friends.

CONSIDERATIONS WHEN USING DIFFUSERS AROUND PETS

- **Nebulizing diffusers or those that diffuse oil directly from the bottle.** Only use open room diffusion if the animal can come in and out of the room. Limit exposure to thirty minutes at a time.
- **Water diffusion.** This is highly recommended with any animal and the best way to begin introducing essential oils into your home. Start with one or two drops of oil in your diffuser per 100 ml water and slowly build your way up to five or six drops. You can also use water diffusion in different ways—in an open room, a closed room, near your animal in a smaller space such as a cage or enclosure, or even via "tenting" (pouring simmering water and essential oils into a glass or stainless bowl, then placing a towel over your head and leaning over the bowl to bask in the aromatic steam) for short periods of time. The latter method allows you to minimize pets' exposure to oils.

With any type of diffusion, monitor your pet's behavior during use and respond accordingly.

HOW TO ADMINISTER ESSENTIAL OILS TO ANIMALS TOPICALLY

Just as any changes you make to your pet's diet need to be done slowly, essential oils should be introduced slowly as well. Start with a small amount of a diluted essential oil (0.5%–1%) and observe your animal's behavior. If the response is neutral but you are not getting the therapeutic effect desired, you can always add more essential oil or increase the frequency of application, but you do not want to start out with a large amount right from the get-go.

- **Applying to paws.** This is not always well tolerated by small animals. Be sure to get the oil on the skin between the paw pads. This is a fairly sensitive area, so be sure to dilute down to 0.5%–1%.
- **DIY.** Adding a couple drops of essential oils to topical products such as shampoo or coconut oil works great. Try out the two DIY pet-friendly recipes on page 185!
- **Applying to ears.** Some animals tolerate having diluted oil applied to the tips of the ears, but many do not. Avoid using this type of application with long-eared dogs as they may shake their head and accidentally get the oil in their eyes.
- **Indirect application.** Apply to bedding or an area your animal frequently comes into contact with.
- **The hooves of large animals.** You can apply oils to where the hoof meets the skin, or the coronet band. This is very helpful when treating foot conditions or lameness in horses.
- **Along the spine.** This is the most common area I use for topical application, as it's the best tolerated.
- **Water misting.** This is great for birds. Add a drop of essential oil to several ounces of water, shake, and spritz on the animal, taking care to avoid the face so the oils don't get in her eyes, nose, or mouth. If your pet seems agitated, use lavender. If she is sluggish, use an uplifting citrus oil. This is also helpful for large animals if you are trying to cover a large area or they don't tolerate regular handling.

For some extra healing, try the Hot Spot Spray (page 186) from Dr. Roark on your animals next time they get a small (or deep) wound.

PET SHAMPOO

This shampoo works great to clean, heal, and restore your pet's fur and skin!

1 cup rolled oats
1½ cups warm distilled water
1 drop lavender essential oil
1½ teaspoons vitamin E oil
1½ teaspoons carrier oil (Mama Z's Oil Base, page 43, works great!)
1 organic green tea bag

SUPPLIES
Blender
Medium glass bowl
Glass jar

1. Mix the oats and water in a blender until smooth.
2. Mix the lavender oil, vitamin E, and carrier oil in a glass bowl.
3. Add the oats to the bowl and mix well.
4. Empty the contents of the green tea bag into your shampoo mix and stir until well blended.
5. Store in a glass jar.
6. Use once a month or more often, preferably immediately following grooming.

DRY SHAMPOO FOR DOGS

For those times when you don't want to give a full bath.

½ cup baking soda
½ cup cornstarch or arrowroot powder

3 drops lemongrass essential oil
3 drops lavender essential oil

SUPPLIES
Glass jar with shaker lid

1. Combine the baking soda and cornstarch or arrowroot powder in the glass jar.

2. Drop the essential oils into the powder mix and shake well.

3. Sprinkle the dry shampoo on your dog, starting at the neck and being careful to avoid the eyes.

4. Work your way down the dog's entire body and thoroughly rub into the fur.

5. Let your dog shake off the excess; then groom her with a dog comb or brush.

HOT SPOT SPRAY

I've seen some before-and-after pictures of a black lab with a huge gash from a dog bite, and this formula worked wonderfully!

10 drops frankincense essential oil
10 drops lavender essential oil
10 drops myrrh essential oil
1 teaspoon colloidal silver
Aloe vera gel

SUPPLIES
2-ounce spray bottle

1. Pour the essential oils and colloidal silver into the bottle.

2. Top off with aloe vera to fill the bottle and shake vigorously.

3. Spray the wound every 2 to 3 hours or as needed to promote healing.

4. Store in the fridge.

HOW TO ADMINISTER ESSENTIAL OILS TO ANIMALS INTERNALLY

It's important to keep in mind that with animals that groom frequently, such as cats, birds, dogs, rabbits, and chinchillas, topical application also means internal application. When applying essential oils topically, be sure to always dilute oils in a vegetable oil such as fractionated coconut oil. Here are some guidelines for safe internal use:

- **Drinking water.** One drop per 2 cups drinking water for dogs; 1 drop per liter for birds and smaller animals. NOT recommended for cats.
- **Food:** One drop per meal, usually in wet food.
- **Doggy toothpaste.** Another great, safe way for your dog to enjoy the therapeutic effects of essential oils is to brush their teeth with the following toothpaste recipe that Dr. Roark created!

K-9 TOOTHPASTE

More than just a breath freshener, this recipe offers healing benefits that help prevent tooth decay!

1 tablespoon bentonite clay
1 tablespoon baking soda
1 or 2 drops peppermint essential oil
Organic, unrefined coconut oil (melted)

SUPPLIES
Glass jar

1. Mix the clay, baking soda, and peppermint in a glass jar.
2. Add enough coconut oil to make a paste.
3. Use a dab to brush your dog's teeth daily!

Part 3
Women's Health

Communities and countries and, ultimately, the world, are only as strong as the health of their women.

—MICHELLE OBAMA

Several years ago, my friend Sue started to suffer from uncontrollable weight gain, hair loss, and insomnia. Her doctors put her on Synthroid (levothyroxine sodium tablets) because they noticed that she had low thyroid hormone levels. They lumped her among the millions now diagnosed with "hypothyroidism" and told her she could expect to live the rest of her life on synthetic hormone replacement therapy, which can—and often does—lead to a litany of side effects ranging from irregular heartbeat to osteoporosis.

The drug quickly started to affect Sue's mental and emotional state. She experienced severe mood swings, insomnia, and brain fog. "I started to go crazy," Sue told me. "I couldn't sleep or think and I was feeling horrible."

Sue got to the point where Synthroid was causing so many horrible side effects that she decided to throw the drugs away and detox cold turkey.

Quitting a prescription drug without the guidance of a trained medical professional is never recommended, but Sue's doctor didn't support her desire to get off Synthroid, so she took matters into her own hands.

When Sue asked me for help and listed her litany of symptoms, her lack of sleep set off alarm bells. Knowing how vital rest is for the body, I simply recommended that she diffuse some lavender in her bedroom and apply some lavender to the back of her neck before going to bed that night.

The very next day, Sue called me. She was ecstatic. She told me that she got a full night's rest for the first time in five years. She wanted to know what else she could do to regain control of her health. We discussed an anti-inflammatory diet and I advised her to stay away from common triggers like grains, dairy, and sugar and to start an exercise regimen that she would stick with.

We also discussed a variety of approaches to using essential oils to heal her thyroid and manage the other symptoms she was battling. I advised her to start applying diluted frankincense essential oil over her thyroid gland to treat her hypothyroidism. We also talked about applying geranium, cilantro, and tangerine oils over the small of her back for adrenal support to help manage her stress response.

Over the next several weeks Sue's symptoms steadily improved. She lost weight, the brain fog vanished, she enjoyed rejuvenating sleep every night, and her hair not only stopped falling out, it started to thicken! Sue even told me that her vision was improving! Her bifocals prescription went from 3.5x to 2.0x after she started applying a mixture of diluted frankincense, helichrysum, lavender, and myrrh around her eye sockets after reading some testimonials online from trusted resources about the ability of these oils to improve vision.

Sue literally transformed her health within weeks of using essential oils and modifying her diet. Her story is what I'd call an unqualified success—and she is just one of many women I've heard from who are experiencing the same healing of their thyroid conditions, seemingly with essential oils.

While thyroid issues are common in women—and may be behind some symptoms that we've come to accept as part of aging, including degrading sleep quality, weight gain, and fatigue—many other symptoms frequently plague women, and essential oils can help with those, too. That's exactly what we'll cover in this section of the book, from premenstrual syndrome all the way through postmenopausal concerns. Essential oils offer rebalancing for women at all phases of their lives.

SPECIAL HEALTH CONSIDERATIONS FOR WOMEN

Did you know that:

- Women enjoy a longer life expectancy, but get sick more often than men.
- Women visit the doctor more often.[1]
- Women experience pain,[2] depression, and anxiety disorders[3] far more often than men.
- Women are more susceptible to poor health outcomes if they have sleep problems than men.[4]

Based on these differences, it would be logical to expect gender-specific treatment from your doctors. Sadly, gender-based health care simply isn't available for the vast majority of people.

Vera Regitz-Zagrosek, director of the Institute of Gender in Medicine at the Charité University Hospital in Berlin, Germany, says:

There is little gender-specific health care; the prevention, management and therapeutic treatment of many common diseases does not reflect the most obvious and most important risk factors for the patient: sex and gender. This omission is holding back more efficient health care, as gender-based prevention measures or therapies are probably more effective than the usual "one-size-fits-all" approach and would benefit patients of both genders.[5]

Aromatherapy, being a female-dominated profession, offers considerably more gender-based recommendations than traditional medicine. However, the research is greatly lacking in this area, and much of the advice is anecdotal—and gender-based aromatherapy research is virtually nonexistent.

We need to take these facts to heart. In spite of knowing that biological and behavioral differences between men and women exist, the drug development process still favors male animals—as many as 90 percent of researchers study male animal models of disease when seeking a cure.[6]

THE BEST ESSENTIAL OILS FOR WOMEN'S HEALTH

It's critical to listen to your body and recognize that you alone know what's best for your health. Health care providers are simply there to help guide you on your journey.

For centuries, women have enjoyed the healing power of essential oils from their favorite plants in the form of salves, anointments, and incense. Now that modern distillation techniques are readily available, we can extract essential oils in their purest, most concentrated form. Women are free to follow their instincts and the advice passed down through the generations to manage their health safely and effectively with essential oils.

Here's the list of specific oils we'll cover in this section:

1. Anise (*Pimpinella anisum*)

2. Basil, sweet (*Ocimum basilicum L*)

3. Clary sage (*Salvia sclarea*)

4. Cypress (*Cupressus sempervirens*)

5. Eucalyptus (*Eucalyptus citriodora, Eucalyptus globulus, Eucalyptus radiata,* and *Eucalyptus tereticornis*)

6. Fennel, sweet (*Foeniculum vulgare*)

7. Geranium rose or rose-scented geranium (*Pelargonium graveolens*)

8. Ginger (*Zingiber officinale*)

9. Grapefruit (*Citrus paradisi*)

10. Lavender (*Lavandula angustifolia*)

11. Marjoram (*Origanum majorana*)

12. Neroli (*Citrus aurantium*)

13. Orange, sweet (*Citrus sinensis*)

14. Peppermint (*Mentha piperita*)

15. Roman chamomile (*Chamaemelum nobile*)

16. Rose (*Rosa damascena*)

17. Sage (*Salvia officinalis*)

18. Tea tree (*Melaleuca alternifolia*)

19. Turmeric (*Curcuma longa*)

20. Vitex (*Vitex agnus-castus*)

21. Ylang Ylang (*Cananga odorata*)

13

Premenstrual Syndrome

I mean if there was any justice in the world you wouldn't even have to go to school
during your period. You'd just stay home for five days and eat chocolate and cry.
—*ANDREA PORTES*, ANATOMY OF A MISFIT

Would you believe me if I told you that PMS wasn't a known health condition until the mid-twentieth century? Evidently, no one knew what was really going on within the female body so no one bothered to give it a medical diagnosis until 1953!

I find this intriguing because women have used natural remedies like herbs and essential oils for centuries to manage symptoms related to their monthly cycle. Yet it wasn't until New York gynecologist Robert Tilden Frank discovered in 1931 that women became "handicapped by premenstrual disturbances" that medical professionals started to take PMS seriously.[1]

Twenty years later, endocrinologists Katharina Dalton and Raymond Greene first coined the term "premenstrual syndrome" in response to recognizing that Dalton's monthly migraines were possibly attributed to low progesterone—the hormone that prepares a woman's body for conception and pregnancy and helps regulate the monthly menstrual cycle. Dalton and Greene published their theory in the *British Medical Journal* in 1953, and the science of PMS was born.[2]

Today, PMS is a household word and receives the attention that it truly deserves in the scientific community. Thankfully, this research includes how to approach PMS more effectively with natural therapies like essential oils!

PMS—FROM IRRITATING TO DEBILITATING

First off, it's important to recognize that horrible PMS doesn't have to be your lot in life. Of course, the mess and hassle of your monthly cycle is unavoidable, but the time leading up to your menses doesn't have to be debilitating or arduous. Just as with cancer, diabetes, heart disease, and most health conditions, it's important to keep these three facts in mind:

1. Most symptoms can be prevented.
2. Your body isn't "drug deficient" and pharmaceuticals are rarely the answer.
3. It takes some trial and error to find the natural remedies that work for your body.

PMS is widespread, occurs naturally, and likely happens due to our lovely little friends called hormones. During your menstrual cycle your hormone levels change, causing a range of symptoms. Finding a way to manage them is a key to providing you with the freedom that you need to enjoy life, no matter the time of the month!

The severity of these symptoms also has a pretty wide range. For some women, PMS symptoms are little more than an annoyance. For others, they can call an immediate halt to your normal routine and make you bedridden for days on end. When PMS is this debilitating, it actually has its own name, premenstrual dysphoric disorder, or PMDD, and it affects up to 8 percent of women worldwide.[3] So if you're feeling like you're completely wiped out by your premenstrual symptoms, you are by no means alone!

The key to determining if you suffer from PMS, PMDD, or something else entirely is whether your symptoms end with your period or continue.

These are the PMS and PMDD symptoms:

- Anxiety
- Breast tenderness
- Bloating
- Depression
- Fatigue
- Headaches and migraines
- Insomnia
- Menstrual cramping
- Mood swings
- Skin breakouts (acne)
- Unhealthy food cravings

As you can imagine, a combination of these symptoms can easily wipe a woman out for days, which is why help is needed. But here's the good news—most, if not all, can be managed with essential oils!

ESSENTIAL OILS FOR PMS

It's important to recognize that no one can completely stop the great hormone shift that happens during the menstrual cycle. That said, it's possible to use essential oils to calm many of the symptoms, so that PMS or PMDD does not have to derail your life every month. Which essential oil is the most effective at treating menstrual cycle–related symptoms? Typically, a combination of oils is the best choice. Here are ten of the more popular essential oils that women use for premenstrual relief today.

1. Lavender

Lavender essential oil is an often-studied oil that has been linked to a number of health benefits, including improved sleep and lowered pain levels. Since many women suffer from menstrual cramps, insomnia, and overall aches and pains, it's a go-to oil during PMS.

Migraines can also be a serious problem when hormones shift during menstruation, and inhaling lavender essential oil has been found in at least one scientifically controlled study to be an effective and safe treatment option to help manage migraines.[4]

Application: Massage a 2%–3% lavender oil dilution into the back of your neck, on your temples, and anywhere else you experience pain or discomfort.

2. Clary Sage

Painful periods, or dysmenorrhea, is one of the most common issues women report and is caused by abnormal uterine contractions. You most likely refer to these as cramps. Long-term use of acetaminophen and nonsteroidal anti-inflammatory drugs

(NSAIDs) like ibuprofen to relieve cramps can have significant consequences (like liver toxicity!), so scientists are trying to find safer alternatives.

In 2012, a fascinating study was conducted in Korea where fifty-five teenage girls were given two different treatments to help with their menstrual pain. One group was given acetaminophen and the other received one ten-minute abdominal massage using essential oils diluted in almond oil. The oils and the ratio of the blend were clary sage, marjoram, cinnamon, ginger, and geranium (1:1:0.5:1.5:1.5), diluted to a 5% concentration. The outcome shouldn't shock us. The aromatherapy group received significantly greater relief than those taking acetaminophen.[5]

Women diagnosed with primary dysmenorrhea found similar relief with a different blend—a 3% dilution of lavender, clary sage, and marjoram blended in a 2:1:1 ratio.[6]

Application: Make my No More Cramps Roll-On and use during your next cycle.

NO MORE CRAMPS ROLL-ON

4 drops ginger essential oil
4 drops geranium essential oil
2 drops clary sage essential oil
2 drops sweet marjoram essential oil
1 drop cinnamon bark essential oil
Almond oil or carrier oil of your choice, as needed

SUPPLIES
10 ml glass roller bottle

1. Drop the essential oils into the roller bottle.
2. Fill the remaining space in the roller bottle with your carrier oil of choice and shake well.
3. Massage over your lower abdomen and small of the back (being sure to cover the ovaries and kidneys) twice daily from the onset of your period until it ends.

3. Fennel

Noting its long history as a natural remedy to regulate menstruation, researchers have been testing fennel's ability to mitigate pain since the turn of the century. One study from 2001 discovered that the essential oil was able to reduce both the frequency and intensity of uterine contractions in rats, which supports why women have traditionally consumed fennel seeds and drunk fennel-infused water during their periods to manage cramps and dysmenorrhea.[7]

Application: Add fennel oil to a topical mixture to reduce cramping.

4. Eucalyptus

Eucalyptus is one of the more popular essential oils available, and for good reason! It can be found in everything from antiseptics to insect repellent. Medicinally it can ease cough and cold symptoms and stimulate the immune system; it has also been shown clinically to be an effective anti-inflammatory analgesic (antipain) agent.[8]

Application: Rub a 2%–3% eucalyptus oil dilution on the abdomen and small of the back to help relieve menstrual cramping.

5. Peppermint

Insomnia and fatigue are difficult to manage, especially for a busy woman who is building her career or raising her family. You don't have time to take a nap simply because it's "that time of the month." Peppermint has an almost instant effect on energy levels, energizing you and giving you the stamina to go about your day. As an added bonus, peppermint has been linked to reduced appetite, so you'll be less likely to give in to those chocolate cravings during PMS.[9]

Application: Use peppermint in your inhaler or diffuser with sweet or wild orange oil for an instant jolt of energy and to reduce unhealthy food cravings and appetite. If you get a hankering for something sweet, try this fast and easy recipe.

SUPERQUICK COCOA MINT DELIGHT

This homemade chocolate candy is superyummy and will help satisfy that sweet tooth in a healthy way!

Serves 1

1 tablespoon unrefined coconut oil
2 teaspoons raw cacao powder
10 drops vanilla-flavored liquid stevia extract
1 drop peppermint essential oil

SUPPLIES
Small glass bowl for mixing
Cupcake liner, muffin tin, or silicone candy mold

1. Mix all the ingredients in a glass bowl until smooth.
2. Pour the mixture into a cupcake liner, muffin tin, or silicone candy mold and refrigerate until hard (about 30 minutes). Enjoy!

→ Watch a video demo of my Superquick Cocoa Mint Delight and learn more about beating food cravings at HealingPowerOfEssentialOils.com.

6. Orange

As a 2014 study out of Japan showed, orange oil is exceptionally effective at boosting mood and creating a more relaxed state of mind.[10] Since women suffering from PMS often feel increased anxiety, stress, and even depression, peace of mind is usually welcomed. From what we can tell, the relaxing prowess of orange oil is best experienced through inhaling the oil, not ingesting it.

Application: Apply a mood-boosting massage oil on the back of your neck, on your wrists, and on the bottoms of your feet at the onset of your period every month.

3 drops opoponax essential oil

3 drops sweet or wild orange essential oil

2 drops frankincense essential oil

2 drops key lime essential oil

2 drops yuzu essential oil

1 ounce carrier oil (we use Mama Z's Oil Base, page 43)

SUPPLIES

Medium glass bowl

Lotion dispenser or glass jar

1. Drop the essential oils into a medium glass bowl.

2. Add the carrier oil and mix.

3. Use as a body moisturizer during your period or rub on your belly, wrists, and temples as needed for an overall emotional pick-me-up.

4. Store in a lotion dispenser or glass jar.

7. Neroli

Also known as "bitter orange," neroli essential oil comes from bitter orange tree blossoms. It has powerful relaxation properties, just like orange; however, it may be especially effective for PMS symptoms because studies have found that it is particularly beneficial when hormones are the trigger for anxiety and stress.[11]

Application: Add 3 drops each of neroli and opoponax to a diffuser to reduce anxiety and stress associated with PMS.

ON-THE-GO ANXIETY INHALER

4 drops neroli essential oil

4 drops opoponax essential oil

4 drops frankincense essential oil

4 drops Indian sandalwood essential oil

SUPPLIES

Precut organic cotton pad

Aromatherapy inhaler

1. Place a cotton pad in the inhaler tube.

2. Drop the essential oils directly onto the cotton pad inside the tube. Alternatively, you can drop the essential oils into a glass bowl, roll the cotton pad in the oils to absorb them, and then insert it into the inhaler tube using tweezers.

3. During those stressful moments during your period or during a panic attack, open the inhaler and take a few deep breaths.

8. Ylang Ylang

A healthy sex drive is crucial to any relationship, and your PMS symptoms shouldn't rob you of that! Thankfully, God has blessed us with natural solutions like ylang ylang, long considered to be the go-to aromatherapy aphrodisiac. In Indonesia, ylang ylang oil is used to reduce sexual anxiety, which can be particularly helpful for women battling PMS-related stress.[12]

Application: Try Mama Z's Spice Up Your Love Life Roll-On!

SPICE UP YOUR LOVE LIFE ROLL-ON

3 drops clary sage essential oil

3 drops geranium essential oil

3 drops ylang ylang essential oil

1 drop jasmine essential oil

Carrier oil of choice (jojoba and fractionated coconut oil absorb quickly and work best), as needed

SUPPLIES
10 ml glass roller bottle

1. Drop the essential oils into the roller bottle.
2. Fill the bottle with your carrier oil of choice and shake well.
3. Use as desired—it works great as a perfume, dabbed on the back of your neck or behind the ears, and can be safely applied over genital region to enhance libido.

9. Rose

Rose essential oil is a fantastic multitasker. It not only has been known to help regulate irregular menstrual periods but also supports good uterine health,[13] provides menstrual cramp relief, and has strong antidepressant properties, helping to boost the mood during menstruation.[14]

Application: Inhale rose essential oil and add a few drops to lotions to apply topically to improve several symptoms of PMS.

10. Sweet Marjoram

Finally, consider adding sweet marjoram essential oil to the mix. This go-to pain relief oil will not disappoint you during your monthly cycle. *The Journal of Obstetrics and Gynecology Research* published a study in 2012 that evaluated how forty-eight patients diagnosed with painful menstrual cramps (dysmenorrhea) responded to daily aromatherapy massage. Diluting a blend of lavender, clary sage, and marjoram in a 2:1:1 ratio in an unscented cream at 3% concentration, participants were advised to use the cream daily to massage their lower abdomen from the end of their last menstrual cycle until the beginning of their next cycle. Compared to the control group, which used a synthetic fragrance cream, the women who enjoyed true essential oil therapy reported a "significant decrease" in pain and reduced the number of days they experienced pain by 25 percent![15]

Application: Make marjoram another addition to your PMS-fighting topical blends by trying this cramp-relieving recipe.

CRAMP-RELIEVING ROLL-ON

4 drops lavender essential oil

2 drops clary sage essential oil

2 drops sweet marjoram essential oil

Carrier oil (jojoba and fractionated coconut oil absorb quickly and work best)

SUPPLIES

10 ml glass roller bottle

1. Drop the essential oils into the roller bottle.

2. Fill the bottle with your carrier oil of choice and shake well.

3. Apply over the lower abdomen and small of the back (being sure to cover the ovaries and kidneys) once a day between monthly cycles.

EXPERIMENT TO DISCOVER YOUR OWN BLENDS

Remember, there is significant benefit from blending essential oils. For example, one research study found that 2 drops of lavender, 1 drop of clary sage, and 1 drop of rose mixed in 1 teaspoon of almond oil helped college women suffering from dysmenorrhea "significantly reduce" menstrual cramping.[16]

While this is just one study showing how a specific blend helps to relieve PMS symptoms, there are many other blends that may prove effective for you. Keep experimenting and don't stop until you find the right blend for your unique physiology!

14

Fertility, Pregnancy, Labor, Postpartum, and Nursing

And behold, even your relative Elizabeth has also conceived a son in her old age; and she who was called barren is now in her sixth month. For nothing will be impossible with God.

—LUKE 1:36-37

n biblical times a woman's role in society was so tied to her ability to bear children that she experienced significant disgrace if she was unable to conceive. Like Elizabeth said after the angel visited her to announce the birth of John the Baptist, "This is the way the Lord has dealt with me in the days when He looked with favor upon me, to take away my disgrace among men." (Luke 1:25)

But was it Elizabeth's "fault"? Why was it *her* shame to bear?

For the 15 percent of couples today unable to conceive, blaming yourself or feeling shame is an unfair burden to carry, and my hope and prayer is that you can find peace. It is heart-wrenching enough to have conceiving a child remain elusive without contributing to the pain by blaming yourself or your spouse.

Particularly, my heart goes out to all the ladies out there who are battling what Elizabeth did nearly two thousand years ago, because until recently, infertility has been generally regarded as a women's health issue. Thanks to our recent better understanding of the human body, we have debunked this stigma, as science has shown us that it definitely takes two to tango. It may surprise you to learn that according to the U.S. National Institutes of Health, the cause of infertility is equally distributed: One-third can be linked to female reproductive issues, one-third to male reproductive issues, and the remaining third to unknown factors.[1]

ESSENTIAL OILS FOR INFERTILITY

I've had women, desperate for help, ask me about how to use essential oils to increase their odds of conceiving and avoiding miscarriage, and I'm always at a loss for a definitive answer because the research is so quiet in this area. What really confuses people is that if you search "essential oils for infertility" online, you'll get hundreds of thousands of hits (536,000 at the time I wrote this book, to be exact) linking you to articles that offer all sorts of infertility solutions using essential oils.

Let me be the one to burst the bubble here: Most of the so-called fertility blends and lists of oils you see out there in the blogosphere are nonsense. There is absolutely no scientific evidence suggesting that they really work.

What we *do* know is that stress, diet, comorbidities (other health issues), prescription drugs, prior use of birth control, and a number of other factors can play a role in the fertility of both partners. We also know that oxidative stress is a leading cause of male infertility and antioxidative supplementation produces a significant improvement in sperm motility (how well the sperm are able to move).[2]

Research suggests that, because they are rich in antioxidants, some essential oils can help, but this is still experimental at best. One review of seven studies assessing the effectiveness of the antioxidant-rich *Satureja khuzestanica* essential oil found that it displays significant antioxidant activity, and that when administered to male rats, it improved sperm quality and litter size.[3]

You've probably not been introduced to this oil yet because it's not readily available for sale to most consumers. Native to southern Iran, *Satureja khuzestanica* is best known in the Middle East for its pain-killing and infection-fighting prowess.

So far in this book, I've tried my best to talk only about essential oils that you can easily purchase, but I'm making an exception for *Satureja khuzestanica*, which is rich in carvacrol and thymol. It's a genus of the *Lamiaceae* family and is related to oregano and thyme—also rich in carvacrol and thymol, respectively.

This is not to say that oral doses of oregano and thyme will get you pregnant. I'm just throwing it out there in case you're interested in trying something a little unconventional—such as taking a drop each of oregano and thyme oil in a gel capsule once a day for three to four weeks to see what happens.

For Women

Of the infertility cases linked to women's health, "bad eggs" are suspected to be a primary cause. This is related to diminished ovarian reserve (DOR), which is when the ovaries lose their normal reproductive potential, thus compromising fertility. "Bad eggs" can be difficult to diagnose and are often overlooked by gynecologists. That said, we do know that while DOR can result from disease or injury, it is generally just a normal result of aging.

When it comes to situations like these, the best solution that I have found is to create a healthy environment in the body and focus on balanced body chemistry. Remember, the real power of essential oils is to help the body reach harmony, and using essential oils known to help the body reach homeostasis can do wonders!

If you're struggling to conceive, try applying a 3%–5% dilution of a known harmonizer such as ylang ylang over your abdomen daily for three to four weeks and see if that can restore the hormonal balance that promotes fertility. Or try the harmonizing blend that follows.

Whatever course you choose, never lose hope. Keep trying different options, and I pray that you find the answer that you're looking for!

Just do me a favor and keep me posted. I always love to read the "medical miracles" that flow through my inbox telling me how essential oils have changed people's lives! My contact information is in the resources section at the end of the book and I'd love to stay in touch.

HARMONIZING MASSAGE OIL

15 drops ylang ylang essential oil

10 drops sandalwood essential oil

10 drops clary sage essential oil

10 drops lavender essential oil

2 ounces evening primrose oil

SUPPLIES

2-ounce glass jar

1. Mix the essential oils in a glass jar.
2. Fill with evening primrose oil and shake gently to mix.
3. Massage over the ovaries twice a day for one month.

ESSENTIAL OILS TO ENHANCE YOUR PREGNANCY

When Mama Z was pregnant with our first baby, she made the decision to give birth at home. Sabrina quickly realized that she was going to need a little extra help, so she contacted some key people in her support group. The point woman was her mom's good friend and prayer warrior Sherryl Buck, aka "Mrs. B." You may recall that Mrs. B helped heal Sabrina's burn when she used a toxic facial cleanser as a teenager.

While they were strategizing in preparation for the upcoming birth, Sabrina asked Mrs. B to come up with an aromatherapy birthing kit. It has carried Mama Z through all four of our home births.

Preparation Breeds Empowerment

The key to Mrs. B's protocol expands well beyond the physiological benefits of using essential oils. Having it at the ready provided Sabrina with pure empowerment, which is something that I believe to be grossly lacking during a vast majority of pregnancies and birthing experiences today. What's more, the chemical compounds in essential oils can greatly reduce the pain, stress, and anxiety that most women experience during birth. In fact, they can even help (safely) speed up the labor process.

Without fail, every time Mama Z and I share our home birth experiences with people, we hear from women that they don't think they have what it takes. "Wow, that's amazing," they invariably say. "I could never do that."

But nothing could be further from the truth!

If you are pregnant and nervous about labor and delivery, no matter where you plan to do it, I want you to know that you do have what it takes! You were made for this!

But if you still feel that you need a little help, I have found that using aromatherapy and other natural tools will give you a tangible reminder that you don't have to be afraid of labor. Using essential oils can help you walk into your birth experience with confidence.

Key Essential Oils for Pregnancy and Labor

Aromatherapy use in midwifery is becoming a popular topic in the research community. And for good reason! Mama Z's story is not an anomaly; women have used plant-based therapies to successfully deliver their babies for thousands of years.

The research suggests that essential oils are a cost-effective approach to help strengthen contractions, speed delivery, and minimize labor pains with virtually no side effects if used properly. They can also help relieve stress and anxiety and decrease nausea and vomiting. An evaluation of 8,058 mothers over eight years confirmed essential oils' ability to minimize labor pains, finding that the use of pethidine (a synthetic opioid pain medication more commonly known as Demerol) decreased from 6 percent to 0.2 percent of the women![4]

If you're worried about baby, don't be. Studies have shown that the number of infants hospitalized in the NICU is significantly lower for women enjoying aromatherapy during labor, which further supports that using essential oils during labor is quite safe and effective.[5]

Of the essential oils to use during pregnancy and labor, the following nine are the most effective.

1 and 2. Clary Sage and Roman Chamomile

Another helpful finding from the study of 8,058 mothers just mentioned is that a 1% topical solution of clary sage and Roman chamomile is one of the most promising aromatic techniques to help relieve labor pain.[6]

Application: Rub a 1%–2% clary sage and Roman chamomile oil dilution on the abdomen and small of the back to help relieve labor pains.

3 and 4. Neroli and Orange

Having a long history of use as an antidepressant, aphrodisiac, and antiseptic, neroli oil is also exceptionally helpful for reducing labor pain. During a very interesting research study conducted in Iran, a group of 126 women in active labor were subject to two different interventions. Women in one group had fresh gauze soaked with neroli distillated water attached to the collar of their gown every thirty minutes. The other group had a similar gauze applied to their collar, but this was soaked only with water, no essential oils. The women's pain was measured when they were dilated at 3 to 4, 5 to 7, and 8 to 10 centimeters.[7]

First off, you've got to tip your hat to these women for not only being willing to participate in a study like this, but also having the mental capacity to concentrate on providing a pain score as they progressed during labor. Truly impressive!

Second, I try not to geek out over numbers and data too much, but bear with me on this one because the following chart paints a picture of how powerful essential oil can be. Think in terms of 0 being no pain and 10 being the worst pain imaginable.

DILATATION STAGES	PAIN (EO GROUP)	PAIN (CONTROL GROUP)
Before Intervention	7.38	7.52
3 to 4 cm dilation	4.97	8.08
5 to 7 cm dilation	6.65	8.67
8 to 10 cm dilation	7.57	9.46

The results came back with a resounding affirmation that simply inhaling neroli essential oil can significantly lessen labor pain and make the birthing process much more enjoyable. Of course, no one is saying that essential oils can make labor and delivery a walk in the park, but the data is telling:

- The average pain the women in both groups experienced was nearly identical before they started the different interventions.

- At early-stage labor (dilated 3–4 cm), the pain the essential oil group experienced was nearly 40% less than that of the women in the non-essential oil group. Offer any woman in labor the opportunity to reduce her pain by 40% and see what she says!
- Women in the essential oil group experienced 25% less pain than the control group during the mid-labor phase (5–7 cm dilation).
- Women in the essential oil group reported experiencing 20% less pain during the final stage of labor (8–10 cm dilation) than the women in the non–essential oil group.

The remarkable thing is that the women who enjoyed the healing benefits of neroli essential oil reported less pain at end-stage labor than women who didn't experience aromatherapy at early-stage labor! And these findings aren't isolated to neroli. Similar results have been found with orange.[8]

Application: Put 3 drops each of orange and neroli in your diffuser at the onset of labor.

5. Geranium

Known for its use in perfume and skin care, geranium oil was evaluated in an Iranian study as a noninvasive treatment for stress during labor. In the study, researchers uncovered that attaching a piece of fabric with 2 drops of geranium onto the patient's collar resulted in decreased blood pressure, pulse rate, and anxiety levels during labor contractions.[9]

Application: Add a drop or two of geranium oil into your diffuser mix during labor. If you don't have a diffuser or the hospital won't permit it, then attach a small geranium-soaked piece of cloth to your gown.

6. Rose

A biblical flower regarded by Muslims as the flower of the prophet Mohammed, *Rosa damascena* is widely used throughout the Middle East and is cultivated for perfume, medicine, and food. Throughout the centuries, women have used rose oil for a number of health concerns, as it is one of the most powerful essential oils for women's health.

Of particular interest for pregnant women is rose's effectiveness in managing anxiety during labor. In 2014, the *Iran Red Crescent Medical Journal* published a research study that randomly assigned 120 first-time moms into two groups—one group received an aromatherapy session and warm foot bath with rose oil at the onset of active and transitional phases of labor, while the other group received a warm foot bath with plain water. The essential oil group reported significantly lower anxiety levels.[10] This reduction in anxiety is a benefit both to the women and to their fetuses.

Application: Spray the Active Stage of Labor Spritzer (page 216) into the air as desired throughout labor.

7. Lavender

Lavender is not just for home-birthers like Mama Z. According to a recent review of the literature, lavender oils have been reported to be particularly helpful at reducing pain in the hospital setting among women who experienced cesarean delivery, episiotomy, or perineal discomfort following vaginal birth.[11]

Application: Have the Early, Active, and Transition Stage of Labor Spritzers (pages 215 and 216) on hand and spray into the air as desired throughout labor.

8. Sage

In several aromatherapy circles, use of sage oil in pregnant women is discouraged. However, a 156-person study published in 2014 found that using a sage incense mask for fifteen minutes during labor worked to significantly decrease pain and shorten delivery times.[12] As I mentioned above, the key here is dosage. Straight sage oil is too concentrated to be considered safe for pregnant women, whereas the hydrosol can do the trick.

Application: Make a sage hydrosol (page 22) spritzer and use as desired.

9. Lemon

Kick morning sickness to the curb! Lemon essential oil can help: According to research, up to 40 percent of women have used some sort of lemon scent to relieve nausea and vomiting, and more than 25 percent of those who have used it reported it as an effective way to control their symptoms.[13] In 2014, a study conducted in Iran set out to test this in the clinical setting to determine if lemon could indeed help pregnant women manage nausea and vomiting. This was actually the first study of its kind conducted on pregnant women, not mice or rats.

The test was simple: to compare how women experiencing nausea and vomiting during their pregnancy responded to either immediately smelling lemon oil or a placebo. When they felt nauseated they were instructed to simply place 2 drops of a solution of lemon oil and almond oil on cotton balls and take three deep breaths through the nose with the cotton 3 millimeters from their face. If necessary, they repeated this simple procedure five minutes later. Half of the women enjoyed a significant decrease in nausea and vomiting, and their symptoms steadily improved by the time the four-day study ended.[14]

NAUSEA-FREE PREGNANCY INHALER

Store this in your purse so you can reach for it whenever you feel nauseated, and be sure to have one handy at work.

15 to 20 drops lemon essential oil

SUPPLIES
Precut organic cotton pad
Aromatherapy inhaler

1. Place a cotton pad in the inhaler tube.
2. Drop the essential oils directly onto the cotton pad inside the tube. Alternatively, you can drop the essential oils into a glass bowl, roll the cotton pad in the oils to absorb them, and then insert it into the inhaler tube using tweezers.

3. When you feel nauseated or like you may vomit, open the inhaler and take a few deep breaths.

➡️ To watch me and Mama Z make this Nausea-Free Pregnancy Inhaler and to learn more about beating morning sickness with essential oils, go to HealingPowerOfEssentialOils.com.

Special Synergy Blend

When it comes to essential oils, using one is good and using a well-chosen few can be even better! In 2003, Korean researchers set out to determine if certain synergies exist among the oils that have traditionally been found helpful for pregnancy. The study compared a group of laboring women who enjoyed an aromatherapy massage (using a 1.5% dilution of clary sage, geranium, jasmine, and rose essential oils) on their back every two hours to a group of women who received no special intervention. They discovered that this special blend had a profound effect at shortening the first stage of labor.[15]

If you or a loved one is pregnant, do them a favor and make this Speedy Delivery Massage Oil blend to help move along the process!

SPEEDY DELIVERY MASSAGE OIL

6 drops clary sage essential oil

6 drops geranium essential oil

3 drops jasmine essential oil

3 drops rose essential oil

2 ounces fractionated coconut, jojoba, or almond oil (or a combination)

SUPPLIES

Glass jar or lotion dispenser

1. Mix the essential oils in a glass container.
2. Fill the container with a carrier oil.

3. Massage over the small of the back every 2 hours from the time labor begins until the transition stage.

Mrs. B's Protocol for Labor and Delivery

My personal favorites are the Early and Active Stages of Labor Spritzers, and I asked Sabrina to make me some for my office. Don't laugh! I know that the kind of labor I put in at my desk is nothing compared to the labor that Sabrina went through to birth our babies. This was years before I really understood the power of essential oils, and I just enjoyed the smell. These blends reminded me of our birth experience together and the courage and strength that I witnessed in my wife. Smell is so powerful and can be used to trigger positive memories and healthy emotions, and I instinctively was drawn to these scents during an exceptionally stressful time in my career.

EARLY STAGE OF LABOR SPRITZER

This spray promotes relaxation, release of fear, clarity of mind, and a state of calm.

3 drops lavender essential oil
3 drops neroli essential oil
3 drops palmarosa essential oil
10 drops organic grain alcohol (190 proof)
10 drops witch hazel
Distilled water, as needed

SUPPLIES
1-ounce glass spray bottle

1. Combine the oils, grain alcohol, and witch hazel in the bottle.
2. Fill with distilled water and shake gently to mix well.
3. Use at the onset of early labor pains by spraying throughout the birthing room.

ACTIVE STAGE OF LABOR SPRITZER

Promotes peace and harmony, release of fear and anxiety, and relaxation.

3 drops lavender essential oil

3 drops neroli essential oil

3 drops rose essential oil

10 drops organic grain alcohol (190 proof)

10 drops witch hazel

Distilled water, as needed

SUPPLIES

1-ounce glass spray bottle

1. Combine the oils, grain alcohol, and witch hazel in the bottle.
2. Fill with distilled water and shake gently to mix well.
3. Use at the onset of active labor by spraying throughout the birthing room.

TRANSITION STAGE OF LABOR SPRITZER

This spray promotes endurance and is energizing.

3 drops lavender essential oil

3 drops clary sage essential oil

3 drops peppermint essential oil

10 drops organic grain alcohol (190 proof)

10 drops witch hazel

Distilled water, as needed

SUPPLIES

1-ounce glass spray bottle

1. Combine the oils, grain alcohol, and witch hazel in the bottle.
2. Fill with distilled water and shake gently to mix well.
3. Use at the onset of the transition stage by spraying throughout the birthing room.

GET READY TO PUSH SPRITZER

This blend promotes courage and is energizing.

3 drops peppermint essential oil
3 drops rosemary essential oil
3 drops eucalyptus essential oil
10 drops organic grain alcohol (190 proof)
10 drops witch hazel
Distilled water, as needed

SUPPLIES
1-ounce glass spray bottle

1. Combine the oils, grain alcohol, and witch hazel in the bottle.
2. Fill with distilled water and shake gently to mix well.
3. Use at the onset of the pushing stage of labor by spraying throughout the birthing room.

Safety Considerations to Keep in Mind

Despite the lack of any conclusive research to suggest that the inhalation, internal, or topical application of essential oils is at all harmful to pregnant women and fetuses, you'll see countless articles online advising against it. The reality is that women have and will continue to use essential oils and plant extracts while pregnant with no adverse effects to their babies.

At this point, I hope that I have established pretty well that, if used properly, essential oils are quite safe and effective to address a number of health concerns. While they rarely have side effects, they still come with inherent risks, and pregnant woman should take great care when using them, just as they would with any natural or medical therapy. Problems can arise when pregnant women use essential oils flippantly, without following basic safety guidelines, or follow misguided advice they read online or hear from someone who lacks experience. Aromatherapists are a good place to start, but we need to remember that even what they recommend is open to debate.

For instance, according to many in the aromatherapist community, pregnant and nursing moms should not use essential oils containing ethers such as fennel and anise. Also, because ketones are not easily metabolized by the liver, they can potentially be toxic, and high-ketone oils like sage and hyssop are also not recommended. Let's discuss these briefly.

Fennel

Recently fennel has been charged as dangerous for humans (especially babies) because of the potential carcinogenicity of estragole, a chemical component of fennel essential oil. If you search online, you'll see it included with anise and other oils listed on various do-not-use lists for pregnant women. This is somewhat misleading, particularly if fennel is used in a blend and is diluted by a carrier oil.

According to several Italian researchers, "This allegation does not consider the remedy is prepared as a matrix of substances, and recent research confirms that pure estragole is inactivated by many substances contained in the decoction."[16]

As I've discussed before, we mustn't take individual component studies out of context. Just because estragole has the potential to be carcinogenic doesn't mean that essential oils containing estragole are necessarily dangerous—that depends on how the remaining chemical compounds within the essential oil itself and the carrier it's mixed in interact with each other.

What this means is that these arbitrary online lists report only part of the story, and this bothers me to no end because they scare many well-intentioned essential oil lovers from using precious healing oils!

Anise

Anise oil got a bad rap when two breastfed infants were hospitalized for a reported lack of weight gain, difficulty feeding, and a number of other alarming symptoms in 1994. Because the mothers of both children had been drinking an exorbitant amount of an herbal tea mixture that contained licorice, fennel, anise, and goat's rue to stimulate lactation (two liters each day), researchers blamed the anethole levels in anise. As a result, anise has been pretty demonized.

Keep in mind that this conclusion was made without even measuring the anethole levels in the women's breast milk or testing the teas for their content—essentially, making a premature judgment based on partial evidence.[17]

I believe this is yet another misguided, non-evidence-based recommendation against using essential oils. Other than these two reports, I don't see any cause for concern—as long as you heavily dilute (1% or lower). Regarding tea, there are such minuscule amounts of essential oils in each cup that there's no concern at all. Of course, it goes without saying that you need to be cognizant of your body. Discontinue use immediately and consult your health care provider if adverse reactions occur.

Sage, Hyssop, and Jasmine

Personally, I don't see the point of incorporating hyssop into any pregnancy protocol because of the potential for it to act as a convulsant (producing sudden and involuntary muscle contractions). Although there is no evidence in the literature that it is a uterine stimulant or abortifacient, it would be wise to avoid it completely during pregnancy. When it comes to sage, however, the issue seems to be dosage, instead of avoiding it by default.

One systematic study I found reported that sage and jasmine can actually increase the level of oxytocin as an effective way to initiate labor, which can be very useful. This is why these oils are used in pregnancies that have gone past their due date. However, their overuse may result in uterus hypertonicity and fetal distress.[18] Again, the key here is dosage, which is a reoccurring theme I have discovered that has helped me navigate through the muddy waters of what the research literature says versus what is used in clinical practice.

The take-home message is that you want to avoid all internal use of sage and jasmine, and keep in mind that high topical and aromatic dosages can stimulate labor.

In addition, here's a list of oils to stay away from that I adapted from the National Association of Holistic Aromatherapists (NAHA).[19] Remember, there are dozens of alternatives to these oils.

ESSENTIAL OILS TO AVOID DURING PREGNANCY

ESSENTIAL OIL	LATIN NAME
Birch	*Betula lenta*
Camphor	*Cinnamomum camphora*
Mugwort	*Artemisia vulgaris*
Parsley seed or leaf	*Petroselinum sativum*
Pennyroyal	*Mentha pulegium*
Tansy	*Tanacetum vulgare*
Tarragon	*Artemisia dracunculus*
Thuja	*Thuja occidentalis*
Wintergreen	*Gaultheria procumbens*
Wormwood	*Artemisia absinthium*

Take-home message: As with any supplement or pharmaceutical intervention, don't believe everything that you read on Dr. Google. Be sure that you're not led by fear, but guided by evidence-based information. This will empower you to take control of your health and the health of your family in a way that honors your faith! Specifically, here are the guidelines to consider:

- Use essential oils the right way by following the safety precautions you've learned in this book, including proper dilution and shelf life.
- Take into consideration centuries of traditional herbal use. WWGGD, right? What Would Your Great-Grandma Do?
- Don't make fear-based decisions.
- Always discontinue any pharmaceutical (with the guidance of your physician or other health care professional) or natural intervention that causes adverse reactions and consult with your health care provider immediately.

With all this said, there are still more safety tips we need to consider, but first let's discuss the key essential oils for labor and nursing.

Vaginal Care

Last but not least on the list of labor and delivery care priorities is to heal and moisturize the perineum, especially if you have an episiotomy or tear. Traditionally, midwives would recommend a concoction of garlic and dried herbs such as comfrey, yarrow, and shepherd's purse in a warm bath after delivery to stimulate healing, prevent infection, and reduce inflammation. Just ask Mama Z and she'll tell you that her meal of gluten-free blueberry pancakes eaten while soaking in an herbal bath was the highlight of the birth. (After baby was delivered, of course!)

Alternatively, an aromatherapy sitz bath would work as well. In 2004, Korean researchers evaluated how sitz bath and soap application using essential oils of lavender, myrrh, neroli, rose, grapefruit, mandarin, orange, and Roman chamomile helped postpartum mothers who delivered vaginally with an episiotomy. They found that both the aromatherapy sitz bath and the soap helped heal the perineum.[20]

To speed up healing after birth, or after any perineum trauma, try these recipes.

AFTER-BIRTH SITZ BATH
Makes 1 bath

1 cup Epsom salts
1 ounce evening primrose oil
1 ounce jojoba oil
1 ounce Dr. Bronner's unscented liquid castile soap
1 drop lavender essential oil
1 drop Roman chamomile essential oil
Hot water, as needed

SUPPLIES
Medium glass bowl

1. Pour the Epsom salts into a bowl. Stir in the carrier oils and soap until evenly distributed.

2. Add the essential oils and mix well.
3. Add just enough hot water to dissolve the mixture.
4. Fill the tub with 4 or 5 inches of warm water, making sure it's not too hot for your bottom.
5. Add the dissolved Epsom salts and oil mixture.
6. Sit in the mixture so the perineum is covered, and soak for 15 to 20 minutes.
7. Be sure to rinse both yourself and the tub afterward.
8. Try to do this every day for the first week postpartum.

PERINEUM HEALING SOAP

When it comes to the all-too-common vaginal dryness that can follow birth, making your own essential oil–based lubricant can do wonders. Being prepared in this area will make all the difference in the world during postpartum sexual intercourse. To learn more about vaginal dryness and to find my Gentle Vaginal Lubricant recipe, go to chapter 17 where I discuss this in more detail.

¼ **cup distilled water**
¼ **cup Dr. Bronner's liquid castile soap**
1 **tablespoon evening primrose oil**
1 **tablespoon jojoba oil**
1 **teaspoon vitamin E oil**
3 **drops grapefruit essential oil**
3 **drops lavender essential oil**
3 **drops myrrh essential oil**
3 **drops neroli essential oil**
3 **drops sweet or wild orange essential oil**
3 **drops Roman chamomile essential oil**
3 **drops rose essential oil**

SUPPLIES
Plastic foaming soap dispenser (glass is best, but since this will be in the shower, it's better to be safe than sorry in case the bottle drops!)

1. Mix the water and liquid soap directly in the soap dispenser.
2. Add the evening primrose oil, jojoba, vitamin E, and essential oils.
3. Secure the pump and shake well.
4. Use as a feminine wash every day for the first month postpartum.

ESSENTIAL OILS FOR NURSING

Mama Z used essential oils extensively to help increase milk production and she has also been a lactation consultant for many years, so this is familiar territory for us.

The research on essential oils and human breast milk production is virtually nonexistent, so Sabrina focused on more traditional herbal preparations. Somewhat unexpectedly, she quickly discovered that the oils extracted from these herbs were even more helpful than the herb itself! These DIY recipes were her mainstay, and still are as she's currently nursing Baby Z number four as I write this!

MAMA'S NEW MILK BODY LOTION

To help prep your body for the milk supply that your baby will need, apply this lotion after you shower when your skin is soft and your pores are open. This is actually part of Mama Z's morning ritual and it has worked like a charm!

8 drops jasmine essential oil
7 drops clary sage essential oil
1 teaspoon vitamin E oil
1 teaspoon aloe vera gel
2 ounces carrier oil or Mama Z's Oil Base (page 43)

SUPPLIES
Medium glass bowl
Lotion dispenser or glass jar

1. Drop the essential oils into a bowl.
2. Add the vitamin E, aloe vera, carrier oil or Mama Z's base, and mix well.

3. Store in a lotion dispenser or glass jar and use daily during the third trimester to help build a milk supply for your baby.

ON-THE-GO MAMA'S MILK-BOOSTING ROLL-ON

5 drops clary sage essential oil
5 drops jasmine essential oil
Carrier oil of choice (jojoba and fractionated coconut oil absorb quickly and work best), as needed

SUPPLIES
10 ml glass roller bottle

1. Drop the essential oils into the roller bottle.
2. Fill the bottle with your carrier oil and shake well.
3. Apply around the breasts in a circular motion and into the armpits two or three times per day, starting in the third trimester.

AFTER LABOR MILK SUPPLY ROLL-ON

After the baby comes, this recipe will help maintain a healthy supply of milk.

5 drops basil essential oil
5 drops fennel essential oil
Carrier oil of choice (jojoba and fractionated coconut oil absorb quickly and work best)

SUPPLIES
10 ml glass roller bottle

1. Drop the essential oils into the roller bottle.
2. Fill the bottle with your carrier oil and shake well.
3. Apply around the breasts in a circular motion and into the armpits two or three times per day.

Safety Considerations

Refer back to the note on page 220 for essential oils that pregnant and nursing moms should approach with caution.

ESSENTIAL OILS FOR POSTPARTUM SUPPORT

"Baby blues" and postpartum depression are serious conditions, and my heart goes out to any woman who has suffered from either. By definition, the "baby blues" only last from a few days to two weeks after birth. Symptoms include:

- Anxiety and feeling overwhelmed
- Brain fog and trouble concentrating
- Depression and a feeling of sadness
- Emotional outbursts and crying
- Hunger and appetite issues
- Mood swings and irritability

More intense by definition, postpartum depression is a proper diagnosis if these issues persist for more than two weeks. I don't feel postpartum depression has received the attention that it deserves in the public health world. It has been reported that one in seven mothers are affected, but that number is likely much higher.[21] There is a gross lack of proper diagnosis as too many women are embarrassed to admit they feel bad after what's supposed to be the happiest moment of their lives.

USING ESSENTIAL OILS AFTER BIRTH

I thank God that my wife hasn't had to deal with postpartum depression, as it does run in her family. It's been such a concern for us that I've prayed specifically about it during all four pregnancies, and she has always been careful to have an ample supply of a special joy-inducing body lotion to use before and after the birth. She wanted something that both she and our babies could enjoy. As an added bonus, it also works wonders at keeping stretch marks away. This is hands down one of my favorite blends that we continue to love to this day. And you don't have to be pregnant, a mother, or even a woman to use it.

This stuff is power in a bottle! It smells good, it works, and people rave about it. Now you can create your own!

If you're pregnant, be sure to have something like this on hand. If you know someone who is pregnant or if you're going to a baby shower soon, why not make it, wrap it up with a nice bow, and bless your loved one with a homemade gift. I promise you it won't disappoint, and will be the hit of the party!

MAMA Z'S JOYFUL BODY OIL

1 ounce carrier oil (we use Mama Z's Oil Base, page 43)
6 drops sweet or wild orange essential oil
6 drops vanilla extract (can be vanilla absolute)

SUPPLIES
Small glass bowl
2-ounce glass bottle or glass salve jar

1. Mix the ingredients in a glass bowl, making sure the essential oils blend into the carrier thoroughly.
2. Use as a body moisturizer or rub on your belly, wrists, and temples as needed for an overall emotional pick-me-up.
3. Store in a glass container.

Note: *This simple blend has worked well for us, but there is an unlimited number of blends that you can come up with.*

Bonus: HOMEMADE VANILLA EXTRACT

Try making make your own vanilla extract for the Joyful Body Oil; it's supereasy!

2 to 4 vanilla bean pods
3 tablespoons of your favorite carrier oil, rum, or bourbon

SUPPLIES
Small glass jar with lid

1. Slice open the vanilla pods and scrape the seeds into the glass jar.
2. If you're using a carrier oil, pour it over the seeds in the jar. Store at room temperature for at least a week—longer for more fragrance—shaking periodically.
3. If you're using a spirit for your base, add it to the jar and let sit in a dark place for a couple of weeks before use.

➔ To watch me and Mama Z make her Joyful Body Oil and to learn more about beating the baby blues with essential oils, go to HealingPowerOfEssentialOils.com.

15

Candida

The righteous cry, and the Lord hears and delivers them out of all their troubles. The Lord is near to the brokenhearted, and saves those who are crushed in spirit. Many are the afflictions of the righteous, but the Lord delivers him out of them all.

—PSALMS 34:17-19

A few years back, a student approached me at the end of one of my essential oils classes. Aliyah's hands were wrapped in bandages and she hid them carefully, embarrassed about how she looked.

Aliyah told me that every month during her menstrual cycle, her hands broke out in oozing, bleeding sores. From what I could tell, she suffered from a very rare disorder called autoimmune progesterone dermatitis (APD). Still very misunderstood, it is suspected that APD is an aberrant skin response to rising progesterone levels during the premenstrual phase of a woman's cycle that occurs right before the menses. The presentation for each woman is different, but skin rashes of varying degrees seems to be a consistent symptom. As hormone levels ebb and flow, the outbreak usually resolves within a few days of menstruation, only to recur during the next cycle.[1]

Aliyah suffered from a litany of other symptoms: brain fog, thinning hair, adrenal fatigue, chronic fatigue, insomnia, low libido, and compromised gut health, but what really threw me for a loop were the sores on her hands. I had never seen anything like it in my life and, evidently, neither had all of the medical doctors, chiropractors, nutritionists, and functional medicine practitioners she had visited.

Unfortunately for Aliyah, her hands never recovered between cycles, so her only recourse was to wrap her hands in soft bandages nearly every day, unable to even grasp a pencil because of the pain. Also, she was a mother of two very young children, so just think about how this affected her quality of life—changing diapers in excruciating pain, not being able to color with her daughter, and barely able to bathe and get herself ready in the morning.

Aliyah's case could definitely be classified as a medical failure, as none of her medical practitioners knew how to help her. She had had virtually every medical test done that her doctors could think of and was ultimately prescribed countless cortisone creams and supplements, to no avail. Aliyah almost went broke paying for the medical bills, prescriptions, and mass amounts of supplements she was taking. Completely strapped for cash, she asked for my recommendation about which one or two essential oils she should try.

When I started to work with Aliyah, the first thing I recommended was that she stop taking all supplements to give her body a break, as the human body cannot thoroughly metabolize all of those ("natural") chemicals, and they end up being excreted through urine and bowel movements. I walked her through a simple, thorough detox to naturally cleanse her gut and to help reset her immune system. There are a variety of strategies that can work in such situations, including monitored water fasts, the Master Cleanse (aka "the lemonade diet"), and simple detox protocols that do not require a massive amount of supplements. Be sure to work with a trained health care professional to develop a detox protocol that works for you. This is not something to undertake without professional guidance, particularly if you suffer from candida overgrowth.

During her cleanse, Aliyah implemented some very strategic and targeted essential oil formulations to facilitate gut health and to boost her immune system. She applied Mama Z's Healing Skin Serum (page 121) topically over her sores, enjoyed a version of my Sleepy-Time Blend (page 50) at night, and carefully consumed antifungal, antioxidant-rich, and anti-inflammatory essential oils.

The results were profound. In fact, Aliyah called it a miracle. Within a couple of weeks her skin condition was completely resolved, and every symptom she suffered from had improved. Aliyah started to sleep better, her sex drive returned, the brain fog disappeared, her hair stopped falling out, she didn't have to consume a pot of coffee to get through the day, and she literally felt like a new woman.

After her cleanse, we implemented an elimination diet where she slowly incorporated safe foods like bone broth and lightly steamed vegetables into her diet while completely omitting all grains, dairy, and sugar.

A COMMONLY HIDDEN INFECTION: CANDIDA OVERGROWTH

In my opinion, the root of Aliyah's problems was an overgrowth of candida—a naturally occurring yeast that resides in your mouth and digestive tract along with billions of other forms of bacteria. Not only did all of Aliyah's symptoms steer me to that conclusion, but her blood results confirmed it. This actually confused her because she hadn't had a yeast infection or other "obvious" signs of too much yeast.

In fact, candida infections (candidiasis) can have three different presentations.[2]

1. **Oropharyngeal candidiasis:** Oral yeast infection, or "thrush"
2. **Vaginal candidiasis:** A vaginal yeast infection
3. **Invasive candidiasis:** A systemic infection where *Candida* species enter the bloodstream (what Aliyah had)

It's important to keep in mind that not all women present candida overgrowth in the same way. Women typically don't go to their doctor unless they get a vaginal yeast infection, which puts them at risk of developing a systemic problem. If you suffer from a combination of the symptoms below, you may have a candida infection:

- Brain fog
- Chronic fatigue
- Foul body odor
- Insomnia
- Low libido
- Sugar cravings
- Seasonal allergies

Vaginal Yeast Infections

Vaginal yeast infections are one of the most common reasons women visit their health care provider. In fact, more than 75 percent of women will suffer from a vaginal yeast infection at least once during their lifetime, and 50 percent will have a recurrent episode.[3] Unfortunately, these numbers are only expected to increase because candida thrives in so many environments:[4]

- Candida thrives in acidic environments.
- Candida feeds on sugar, and flourishes in patients with high-sugar diets and/ or uncontrolled diabetes.
- Candida has a tendency to develop in immune-compromised patients with HIV or who are undergoing chemotherapy.
- Candida is more likely to thrive in individuals who take antibiotics, as the medicine wipes out friendly bacteria as well as pathogenic bacteria; with no friendly bacteria to keep it in check, candida flourishes.
- Candida is triggered by vaginal dryness and tightness during sex.
- Certain strains of candida have developed antifungal drug resistance, making it untreatable in many cases.

Typically experienced as genital itching, burning, and sometimes a thick vaginal discharge that resembles cottage cheese, the symptoms of a yeast infection are similar to other genital infections, so it's important to visit your health care provider if you have any of these symptoms.

In most cases, the infection is caused by the candida that is already living in a woman's body. It is actually quite normal for candida to exist in the mouth, gastrointestinal tract, and vagina without any complications. The problem occurs when something goes awry, such as an increase in vaginal acidity, hormonal imbalance, or undue stress, which compromises the immune system. In some cases, candida infections can be sexually transmitted, but that is rare.

THE PROBLEM WITH ANTIBIOTICS AND ANTIFUNGALS

Urinary tract infections (UTIs) are another common ailment that many women suffer from. The good news is that essential oils are an extremely effective natural therapy for these painful infections. Applying a 5% dilution of traditional antibacterial oils like clove, lemongrass, oregano, and thyme over the abdomen two to three times per day can do a wonderful job stopping the infection.

Sage is also a recommended therapy. In a study comparing basil, lemongrass, and sage essential oils against microorganisms isolated from urinary tract infection, sage exhibited enhanced inhibitory activity with 100% efficiency against *Klebsiella* and *Enterobacter* species, 96% against *Escherichia coli*, 83% against *Proteus mirabilis,* and 75% against *Morganella morganii.*[5]

In a study evaluating *Staphylococcus aureus* and *Escherichia coli* (bacteria that are both known to cause urinary tract infections), palmarosa oil was shown to be an effective remedy.[6]

Unfortunately, rather than targeting UTIs naturally, far too many doctors prescribe antibiotics, which put women at risk of also developing a yeast infection since these drugs destroy key healthy bacteria that protect the vagina from candida overgrowth. Remember, your human body contains approximately 30 trillion bacteria and about 1 quadrillion viruses[7]—you need plenty of friendly bacteria to keep the harmful bacteria in check.

Multidrug-resistant *Candida albicans* is on the rise because antifungal drugs have been overused and are all but useless at resolving the root cause of the infection.[8] Couple this with a highly acidic diet that's rich in sugar, grains, and dairy and the perfect environment for candida outbreaks exists in women all over the world.

To complicate matters, the situation has become somewhat grim because antifungals are known to cause nervous system damage! Even though the FDA has finally issued a warning against using these drugs for "uncomplicated infections,"[9] doctors still do every day. Be sure to question your doctor if she prescribes the following:

- Ciprofloxacin (Cipro)
- Gemifloxacin (Factive)
- Levofloxacin (Levaquin)
- Moxifloxacin (Avelox)
- Norfloxacin (Noroxin)
- Ofloxacin (Floxin)

The solution is simple: Use antibiotics and antifungals only when absolutely necessary. Easier said than done, right? This is where choosing the right health care provider is key. You should be able to work with your doctor to manage simple infections naturally first. Then, if you don't get the results that you're looking for, consider more aggressive measures like drugs.

TOP SEVEN ESSENTIAL OILS FOR CANDIDA

It's important to point out that most of the essential oil recommendations out there for candida focus on treating vaginal infections or thrush, not invasive candidiasis. This is not to say that essential oil protocols are nonexistent for systemic candida overgrowth, but in my opinion you will be better served if you use essential oils in conjunction with significant dietary changes as your first line of defense. This is particularly true if you're trying to treat a vaginal yeast infection or oral thrush.

As with Aliyah's case, I have seen some dramatic results when the following seven essential oils are used to treat candida overgrowth.

1. Tea Tree

By far, the go-to antifungal oil is tea tree. Tea tree has a long history as a skin treatment and air-purifying agent, and has been used with great success to treat fungal infections, especially candida.[10]

Application: Douche up to twice a day to treat a vaginal yeast infection using the following protocol. Similarly, oil pulling with lavender and tea tree can help oral thrush. If in a sexual relationship, make sure your partner is applying a 1% dilution of tea tree body oil over his or her genitals to prevent passing the infection back and forth. As mentioned above, it's rare for candida to be passed between sexual partners, but it's better to be safe than sorry.

Note: Many conventional, store-bought douches are filled with irritant chemicals and artificial fragrances, so I recommend avoiding those. Instead, just get a douche bag and DIY with essential oils.

CANDIDA DOUCHE

2 drops lavender essential oil
2 drops tea tree essential oil
1 teaspoon raw honey
½ cup warm distilled water

SUPPLIES
Small glass bowl
Douche bag (which you can find at most drugstores) or squeeze bottle

1. Mix the essential oils and honey in a glass bowl.
2. Add the water and stir until the honey dissolves.
3. Fill a douche bag with the solution.
4. Sitting on the toilet or squatting in your shower, rinse the vaginal cavity using the douche bag or squeeze bottle.
5. Immediately afterward, wash the vulva with mild soap and water in the shower.
6. Douche once or twice a day for up to two weeks at a time.

Note: *Alternatively, you can try the pessary (vaginal suppository) or tampon approach if you stick with the gentler oils. Do not use thyme, peppermint, lemongrass, or the other more caustic oils (i.e., "hot" oils like cinnamon, clove, and oregano that cause a burning sensation), or you could cause serious discomfort!*

CANDIDA PESSARY

9 drops lavender essential oil

9 drops tea tree essential oil

3 tablespoons unrefined coconut oil or evening primrose oil

2 tablespoons organic plain yogurt (no flavoring, no sugar added)

1 tablespoon raw honey

SUPPLIES

Medium glass bowl

Small round or oval-shaped molds (ice cube trays work great)

Continence pad or panty liner

1. Mix the essential oils, carrier oil, yogurt, and honey in a glass bowl.

2. Pour the mixture into small molds or ice cube trays and freeze overnight.

3. Before bed, insert a cube into the vagina; be sure to wear a pad or panty liner to protect your clothes and sheets.

4. In the morning, clean any excess oil remaining in the vagina with unscented soap and water in the shower.

5. Repeat every night for one week.

CANDIDA TAMPON

I know you'll read a lot of conflicting things out there in the blogosphere about using essential oils in tampons, but let me put your mind to rest. Critical care registered nurse Dr. Jane Buckle, author of *Clinical Aromatherapy: Essential Oils in Healthcare*, states that "tea tree tampons are a very safe and effective method of eradicating candidiasis (and many other vaginal infections), and there appear to be no adverse effects."[11] According to Dr. Buckle, the key is using the right type of Australian tea tree (*Melaleuca alternifolia*), and she claims that it takes only three days for the infection to be removed! Evidently, the other species of tea tree oil don't do the trick.

So, with Dr. Buckle's approval in mind, I present to you a very safe, highly diluted candida tampon recipe.

2 drops lavender essential oil

2 drops tea tree essential oil

½ teaspoon raw honey

2 teaspoons unrefined coconut oil or evening primrose oil

1 teaspoon organic plain yogurt (no flavoring, no sugar added)

SUPPLIES

Medium glass bowl

Cotton tampon (unbleached and organic if possible)

Continence pad or panty liner

Small glass jar for storage

1. Mix the essential oils, honey, coconut oil, and yogurt in a glass bowl.

2. Place the tampon in the mixture for several minutes to absorb the contents. Insert into the vagina before going to bed.

3. Wear a pad or panty liner to absorb the discharge.

4. Remove the tampon first thing in the morning and clean the vagina with plain, unscented soap and water in the shower.

5. Repeat every night for one week.

Note: *Between uses, store the mixture in a small glass jar in your refrigerator. Soften it by immersing the jar in a bowl or pot filled with enough warm water to melt the contents.*

 To watch me and Mama Z make this candida tampon and to learn more about beating yeast fungal infections naturally, go to HealingPowerOfEssentialOils.com.

I can already see the wheels turning in your mind and hear your thoughts. "Dr. Z, didn't you just say sugar feeds candida? Is it safe to use honey?"

Good question!

Eating white processed sugar makes you more susceptible to vaginal infections and other candida outbreaks. Topical application of raw honey is a completely different story. Several research articles and aromatherapy textbooks discuss the antifungal properties of raw honey, especially against candida.[12]

Interestingly, yogurt and honey seem to work synergistically, which is why I have included them in these recipes. A 2015 Iranian study tested this theory and evaluated how seventy women with vaginal infections responded to creams made up of yogurt and honey compared to clotrimazole, a popular antifungal medication. The researchers described the power of the alternative treatment this way: "This study indicated that the therapeutic effects of vaginal cream made up of yogurt and honey is not only similar to clotrimazole vaginal cream but *more effective* in relieving some symptoms of vaginal candidiasis" (emphasis mine).[13]

You'll find similar recipes in standard aromatherapy texts—this approach has been validated and is well worth trying.

2. Lavender

As we have seen, tea tree and lavender work synergistically to combat fungal infections, but don't discount lavender by itself, because it's quite potent! Similar to the study evaluating yogurt and honey, another article published in 2015 compared the use of lavender essential oil to clotrimazole on vaginal candidiasis. Interestingly, during the first forty-eight hours of applying both treatments, clotrimazole had a greater effect than the lavender essential oil on candida in vitro, but after forty-eight hours the results were the same.[14] Natural therapies are not always the fastest solution, but they end up getting the job done as well as the medical alternative if they have enough time.

As it's one of the safest essential oils to use, why not try incorporating lavender into your diet to help battle candida internally? This can be particularly helpful if you suffer from sugar addiction and crave chocolate!

Application: Avoid the excess sugar and additives in store-bought chocolate bars and make your own chocolates at home! Cacao is naturally rich in magnesium, a critical mineral for over five hundred bodily functions, including hormonal balance. A touch of lavender essential oil helps you feel rejuvenated and uplifted, and can even help battle systemic candida overgrowth!

HOMEMADE CHOCOLATE WITH LAVENDER AND GOJI BERRIES

This recipe is courtesy of my good friend Magdalena Wszelaki, founder of HormonesBalance.com and the author of *Cooking for Hormone Balance*.

Makes 24 chocolates

1 cup cocoa butter
1 cup unsweetened cocoa powder
1 teaspoon vanilla extract
8 drops stevia extract
1 drop lavender essential oil
¼ cup raw goji berries

SUPPLIES
Grater
Medium glass or metal bowl
Medium saucepan
Silicone candy mold

1. Grate the cocoa butter into the bowl until it is shredded into small pieces.
2. Pour an inch of water into a saucepan slightly smaller than the bowl's diameter and bring to a simmer. Nestle the bowl into the top of the saucepan, taking care not to let the bottom of the bowl touch the water. (Or, if you have a double boiler, use that!) Stir the cocoa butter until melted. Remove from the heat.
3. Stir in the cocoa powder, vanilla, stevia, and lavender oil. Mix well until the ingredients are incorporated and smooth.
4. Use a spoon to pour the liquid chocolate into a silicone chocolate mold. Top the chocolate with a few goji berries.
5. Let the chocolate firm up for an hour in the refrigerator before removing it from the mold and serving.

3. Thyme

Broad-spectrum antibiotics and antifungals have failed to stop the candida epidemic, so researchers are investigating natural broad-spectrum alternatives, including essential oils. A study out of Poland discovered that both tea tree and thyme oils have the uncanny ability to change the morphology and metabolism of yeast enzymes,[15] suggesting that these essential oils can significantly impact *Candida albicans* pathogenicity and that candida cannot become resistant to these oils.

Application: Make a 2% body oil dilution with thyme and coconut oil and apply over your abdomen to treat systemic candida overgrowth. Not safe for vaginal application.

4. Peppermint

In 2010, one of the most exhaustive studies to date evaluated how thirty different essential oils inhibited the growth of *Candida albicans* in vitro. Of those tested, twelve were found to be ineffective. Eighteen were found to be effective; of these, eucalyptus and peppermint oils stood out. At concentrations as low as 0.15%, both showed significant fungicidal properties.[16]

Application: Try oil pulling with one drop of peppermint to cleanse the mouth of oral thrush. Not safe for vaginal application.

5. Geranium

Specifically testing how geranium helped mice with vaginal candidiasis, researchers discovered that the oil had a minimal effect when applied alone. However, when used in combination with vaginal washing, the infection decreased significantly.[17]

Application: After showering, massage a 1% body oil dilution of geranium oil mixed with a carrier over the genital region to help prevent yeast infections. Coconut and evening primrose oils are the carrier oils of choice.

6. Lemon

Truly a jack-of-all-trades, lemon has performed well against drug-resistant strains of a number of bacteria and fungi, including MRSA and candida.[18] Additionally, multiple commercial lemon oils have been shown to contain a broad-spectrum ability, killing a variety of fungal strains, including *C. albicans*, *C. tropicalis,* and *C. glabrata.*[19] Not all lemon oils are equal in treating candida symptoms, however. Be sure to use those that are rich in monoterpenoids.

The key takeaway from the study is this: Limonene—a monocyclic terpene—is the main ingredient in most lemon essential oils on the market. However, the antifungal activity depends on the content of oxygenated monoterpenes—the higher the content, the better the fungicidal effects that were observed. If you want to battle candida, try to get a chemical analysis of the brand of lemon oil before buying to be sure it contains these constituents. You can usually find this information on the oil manufacturer's website.

ANTIFUNGAL CONSTITUENTS IN LEMON ESSENTIAL OIL

OXYGENATED ALIPHATIC MONOTERPENES	OXYGENATED MONOCYCLIC MONOTERPENES	OXYGENATED BI- AND TRICYCLIC MONOTERPENES
Trans-citral	Trans-geraniol	Verbenol
Cis-citral	Carvone	Pinocarveol
Cis-geraniol	Trans-carveol	trans-verbenol
Linalool	trans-p-2,8-menthadien-1-ol	
	1-terpinen-4-ol	

From M. Białoń et al., "The Influence of Chemical Composition of Commercial Lemon Essential Oils on the Growth of *Candida* Strains," *Mycopathologia* 177, nos. 1–2 (2014): 29–39. DOI: 10.1007/s11046-013-9723-3.

Application: As with lavender, try incorporating lemon essential oil into your culinary creations—it's delicious when stirred into olive oil that you drizzle on salad, for example, mixed into yogurt, or added to guacamole—for an extra antifungal punch. A little goes a long way, so start with one drop and add more to taste.

CANDIDA-SAFE CACAO TRUFFLES

This low-sugar, guilt-free dessert is the perfect blend of sweet and tart for an after-dinner treat. The beet and avocado give the inside filling a smooth and rich texture while providing liver support and a boost of progesterone. The citrus essential oil is rich in d-limonene, a natural liver detoxifier. A truly healing recipe courtesy of Magdalena Wszelaki, founder of HormonesBalance.com and the author of *Cooking for Hormone Balance*.

Makes 10 to 12

2 medium beets

1 large avocado

¼ cup blueberries

¼ cup raspberries

1 teaspoon vanilla extract

3 tablespoons maple syrup

4 drops lemon essential oil

2 cups unsweetened cacao powder

TOPPINGS

Walnuts, finely chopped

Unsweetened coconut flakes

Turmeric powder

Additional cacao powder

SUPPLIES

Medium saucepan

Food processor or blender

1. Fill a medium saucepan with water and bring to a boil. Add the beets and cook until soft, about 40 minutes. Drain.

2. Let the beets cool, then peel and cut into cubes.

3. Combine the beets, avocado, blueberries, raspberries, vanilla, maple syrup, and lemon oil in a food processor or blender and blend until smooth.

4. Pour in the cacao powder ½ cup at a time, blending after each addition, until fully incorporated.

5. Transfer the mixture to a bowl and refrigerate for at least 1 to 2 hours. Refrigerating overnight will make the mixture harder and easier to roll into balls.

6. Scoop spoonfuls of the mixture into your hands and roll into balls about an inch in diameter.

7. Place the toppings of your choice—walnuts, coconut flakes, additional cacao powder, or even turmeric—on a plate and roll the balls to coat.

8. Refrigerate in a covered container until ready to serve.

7. Clove

Rich in eugenol—a chemical component of plants with antiseptic properties—clove oil is a superhero at killing microorganisms. Research has shown that its power against candida strains is so potent that it can reduce the fungi to near zero levels, including fluconazole-resistant strains![20] Before you apply it topically over sensitive areas of your body, however, take great caution and be sure to dilute it properly. I recommend starting at a 1% dilution and working your way up as long as no irritation occurs. Clove is powerful and can seriously aggravate your skin.

Application: Try combating candida internally with these candida capsules.

CANDIDA CAPSULES
Makes 1 application

2 drops clove essential oil
2 drops thyme essential oil
Organic extra-virgin olive oil, grapeseed oil, or unrefined coconut oil (melted)

SUPPLIES
Pipette
Size 00 capsule (time-release capsules are preferable)

1. Using a pipette, drop the essential oils into the narrower, bottom half of the capsule.

2. Fill the remaining space in the capsule with the carrier oil of your choice.

3. Fit the wider, top half of the capsule over the bottom half and secure snugly.
4. Swallow the capsule immediately with water on an empty stomach.
5. Take once or twice daily for fourteen days.

Note: *Do not premake capsules and store for future use because you do not want them to leach or erode.*

BLENDS THAT TAKE AIM AT CANDIDA

In an attempt to determine which oils work best synergistically against microorganisms like candida, researchers are starting to get creative in their testing. For instance, a recent study looked at the effectiveness of two different preparations, and the results showed that lavender, clary sage, and ylang ylang oils exhibited stronger antimicrobial activity than a preparation of petitgrain, clary sage, and jasmine oils.[21] While we're still a long way off from finding that "perfect" blend, this is a great start and I'm glad that scientists are looking this deeply into the chemistry.

CANDIDA SYNERGY BLEND BODY OIL

10 drops clary sage essential oil
10 drops lavender essential oil
10 drops ylang ylang essential oil
1 ounce evening primrose oil
1 ounce organic, unrefined coconut oil

SUPPLIES
Glass jar or lotion dispenser

1. Mix the essential oils, primrose oil, and coconut oil in a glass jar or lotion dispenser.
2. Use as an after-shower body oil to moisturize the skin and combat candida infections.

Keep in mind that as you branch out and expand your medicine cabinet to treat candida, certain oils are inherently safer and more effective than others. For instance, oils rich in oxides have a tendency to irritate already sensitive vaginal tissue.[22] This would include oils rich in both 1,4 and 1,8-cineole, so use caution with the following oils:

- Bay laurel
- Cajuput
- Cardamom
- Eucalyptus (*globulus* and *radiata*)
- Galangal
- Ho leaf
- Myrtle
- Niaouli
- Rosemary (1,8-cineol ct.)
- Sage
- Saro
- Spike lavender

Alternatively, essential oils that contain the following alcohols are much gentler:[23]

- Linalool—clary sage, lavender, lavandin, and ylang ylang
- Borneol—lavandin, lavender, and rosemary
- Geraniol—palmarosa, thyme, and *Melissa*
- Citronellol—rose, geranium, citronella, and *Melissa*
- Menthol—peppermint

As you can see from this exhaustive list of essential oil uses and applications, you have options to treat candida naturally. With that said, if you're on the SAD (Standard American Diet), are on recurring cycles of antibiotics, or are dealing with unresolved chronic stress in your life—all common triggers of candida—then using essential oils to beat yeast infections is like taking one step forward and two steps back.

As with all of the conditions discussed in this book, a completely holistic approach is a must if you want to fully resolve a candida infection. Sure, essential oils can help, but they are only one piece of the (organic, gluten-free, naturally sweetened) pie!

16

Autoimmunity

n my work, I talk to many people about their health. And many of them share tales about their autoimmune conditions, and how they are unable to enjoy life because of the unpleasant and often debilitating side effects of their particular disease.

The many autoimmune patients I have helped all share some basic commonalities:

- People taking immunosuppressive drugs are often restricted in their ability to enjoy life due to unpleasant side effects.
- Their immune systems are wiped out, and they are perpetually trying not to get sick.
- Many live in a constant state of fear, never knowing where the next immune threat will come from.
- They are often apprehensive about the foods that they eat because so many of them develop sensitivities due to their hyperactive immune system.
- Some are hesitant to even go out in public and spend time around other people for fear of being exposed to germs.

To make matters worse, the drugs prescribed to many autoimmune patients are known to increase the risk of cancer, depression, diabetes, infection, kidney failure, intestinal bleeding, muscle loss, and osteoporosis.[1]

BEATING AUTOIMMUNITY GOD'S WAY

And not only this, but we also exult in our tribulations, knowing that tribulation brings about perseverance; and perseverance, proven character; and proven character, hope; and hope does not disappoint, because the love of God has been poured out within our hearts through the Holy Spirit who was given to us.

—Romans 5:3–5

"And hope does not disappoint . . ."

Why some people get sick and others don't, I'll never know.

Maybe the reason so many people suffer from AI conditions is because it's virtually impossible to find pure air, food, and water nowadays. Maybe it's because we live in the most toxic environment the world has ever known, and it's only by the grace of God that we are all not dead at this point. One thing I am quite certain about is that we have been gifted with the remarkable ability to adapt to our surroundings and to heal ourselves under the right conditions, which is why it's so important that we treat our bodies right.

Seeing far too many people lose the mental and emotional battle associated with autoimmune conditions, my suggestion is to recite daily positive affirmations to help maintain a proper mental focus. Remember, your body will follow your thoughts, which means that your health will follow your beliefs. The road is much harder to climb if you resign yourself to being sick instead of keeping faith that you will recover. Make sense?

To see how I recite my favorite healing affirmations and to download a full-color printable PDF to help you proclaim your own affirmations, go to HealingPowerOfEssentialOils.com.

AUTOIMMUNITY 101

Of all the diseases that carry with them the burden of hopelessness, fear, frustration, and utter confusion, autoimmune (AI) conditions are the most insidious. Here's a quick snapshot to explain why: More than 50 million Americans have an autoimmune disorder or disease (more than cancer and heart disease combined)[2]— 80 percent of them women.[3] (We don't know precisely why this is so, but convincing research has found that gender-based differences in gene expression are a likely culprit.)[4] Autoimmunity is the eighth leading cause of death in women (shortening a patient's lifespan by eight years),[5] and creates $120 billion in spending each year, twice the burden of cancer, and is a contributing factor to personal bankruptcy.[6]

There is a strong hereditary component, making AI disorders almost impossible to prevent. The most common form of treatment is prescription immunosuppressants, which make you more susceptible to other diseases.

It's no wonder people with autoimmune issues have a tendency to despair—they are battling a condition that can be defined as "self attacking self," and their only medical hope is to take drugs that dampen their immune system. Unlike cancer, where the enemy is a tumor or malignant cells—or type 2 diabetes, where the enemy is usually lack of exercise and poor food choices—the primary foe in autoimmune disease is your own body! This throws people for a loop and is extremely difficult to process, not only on an emotional level, but spiritually.

That said, I know from the AI patients I've worked with that it is possible to get to the point where you can make progress and peace with your condition. I hope that the following suggestions will help you find acceptance *and* relief from your symptoms!

INFLAMMATION: THE KEY TO REVERSING AUTOIMMUNITY

Autoimmune conditions like rheumatoid arthritis, Crohn's disease, ulcerative colitis, and others are known as *chronic inflammatory diseases* because they take much longer to develop, last more than three months, and present a multitude of lifelong symptoms. Signs that your body may be chronically inflamed include:

- Generally not feeling well
- Exhaustion
- Fever
- Increased metabolism (due to fever)
- Changes in white blood cell count

To put all this into perspective, let's remember that inflammation is not necessarily bad and can be part of your body's healing mechanism. When you injure a muscle (as with a twisted ankle), for example, your immune system initiates an inflammatory response by sending blood and immune cells to the affected area, which can result in redness, heat, and swelling. Otherwise, *why would God design our immune systems to function this way?* The problem is when our bodies become chronically inflamed due to preventable risks like poor food choices, stress, anxiety, and overuse of harmful medications.

Just think about the number of people who currently take prescription and over-the-counter drugs today. Consider how the SAD diet is primarily based on processed and inflammatory foods. It's no wonder that 50 million Americans suffer from autoimmune disorders!

Thankfully, a growing number of physicians are looking into the root causes of disease and are helping their patients get off of unnecessary drugs, discover unknown food allergies, detoxify from heavy metal poisoning, and address other chronic inflammation triggers.

The bottom line is this: If you want to prevent or treat autoimmunity effectively, you need to solve your inflammation problem. In my opinion, you'll get the biggest bang for your buck by working with a skilled health care provider who will help you modify your diet, exercise regularly, and implement a natural remedy protocol including supplements and essential oils.

THE TRUTH ABOUT ESSENTIAL OILS AND AUTOIMMUNITY

If you've been following my work for any length of time, you know that I try not to get stuck in the hype about the power of essential oils. As a trained public health researcher, I'm about as evidence-based as they come, which is why I always take great care to comb through the medical literature and reference scientific studies in my articles and books.

I say this because, contrary to popular belief, there is very little research about how essential oils can affect the root causes of autoimmunity.

You might find this counterintuitive because of the sheer volume of resources that you see in the blogosphere claiming to have definitive answers, but believe me when I tell you that they are just expressing their opinion. And there are a lot of opinions out there! Literally millions of website pages get referenced by Google when you search for topics like "essential oils autoimmune disease," "essential oils for rheumatoid arthritis," "essential oils for multiple sclerosis," and the 120-plus other AI conditions that people suffer from.

This is not to say that all of these websites are publishing nonsense, though many certainly are. The point is to emphasize that we literally have no idea which essential oils are best for specific autoimmune conditions, the dosage at which we should administer them, what the contraindications are, and how to use them safely and effectively to treat autoimmune disease. This is truly uncharted territory in the scientific frontier.

I'm very serious when I say that we are shooting blind here and, because of the risk of adverse drug interactions in addition to counterproductive immune system stimulation, most health care providers have taken a broad-brush approach by recommending against using essential oils altogether. All of this should lead us to use great caution before treating autoimmune conditions with essential oils.

KEY SAFETY CONSIDERATIONS

The traditional aromatherapy recommendation for autoimmune patients is to avoid all immune-stimulating essential oils, which basically limits your choices to just a few because virtually every essential oil stimulates the immune system to some degree. Personally, I think this is a little extreme, and I have seen people (like Sue, who suffered from hypothyroidism and whose story I shared on page 189, and Mary, whom you'll meet in chapter 17, and others that we've talked about in this book) do very well using the essential oils we've discussed so far.

Nonetheless, it is absolutely critical to keep your health care provider in the loop when administering essential oils to treat autoimmune conditions if you're taking immunosuppressant drugs. This is particularly true if you plan to use them internally in capsules, and be extremely careful when incorporating essential oils into your food recipes. Dosage is key and you always want to err on the side of caution. It is much safer to use essential oils topically and in an inhaler.

HOW ESSENTIAL OILS FIT INTO THE AUTOIMMUNE PUZZLE

When it comes to essential oil therapy, I have found that implementing a regimen of anti-inflammatory oils is very helpful because, as we have learned, inflammation is a key trigger. My suggestion would be to incorporate the easy recipes that follow into your daily natural health regimen and see how your body responds. Be sure to let your health care provider know what you're doing and stay current on your blood work and other lab tests to track the results.

The first step is to create an inflammation blend that suits your senses, and we know the main anti-inflammatory components to look for:[7]

- **1,8-Cineole**—found in eucalyptus (*globulus* and *radiata*), niaouli, cajuput, cardamom, rosemary, and sage
- **Anethole**—found in anise, cedarwood, and fennel
- **Borneol**—found in lavender, rosemary, lavandin, spike lavender, and sage
- **Eugenol**—found in clove, black pepper, and basil

In addition to the chemical components above, the following essential oils have been shown to have very promising anti-inflammatory properties according to research studies:

- Caraway[8]
- Clove[9]
- Eucalyptus[10]
- Ginger[11]
- Lavender[12]
- Marjoram[13]
- Oregano[14]
- Peppermint[15]
- Roman chamomile[16]
- Tea tree[17]
- Thyme[18]
- Turmeric[19]

When using these anti-inflammatory oils, you'll more than likely discover that certain blends work better than others.

In 2006, a study conducted at the Royal Adelaide Hospital in South Australia evaluated the anti-inflammatory impact of caraway and peppermint essential oils both individually and blended together compared to a placebo in a group of animals suffering from post-inflammatory visceral hyperalgesia (painful gut inflammation). Interestingly, neither oral peppermint nor caraway treatments for fourteen days were very effective alone at treating the pain or inflammation, but when combined, they reduced the condition by 50 percent![20]

I like this combo because caraway and peppermint are safe oils that are regularly used in capsules for gastrointestinal complaints. Research like this, albeit on animals, is very promising as traditional use supports that these oils could work with humans, too.

Application: Enjoy the anti-inflammatory synergy of caraway and peppermint by trying the body oil and capsule formulations below.

INFLAMMATION-SOOTHING ROLL-ON

5 drops caraway essential oil
5 drops peppermint essential oil
2 drops lavender essential oil
Fractionated coconut oil or the carrier oil of your choice, as needed

SUPPLIES
10 ml glass roller bottle

1. Drop the essential oils into the roller bottle.
2. Fill the remaining space in the bottle with fractionated coconut oil.
3. Massage over your abdomen and the bottoms of your feet twice daily for 2 weeks.

INFLAMMATION-SOOTHING CAPSULES

Makes 1 application

2 drops caraway essential oil

2 drops peppermint essential oil

Organic, extra-virgin olive oil, grapeseed oil, or unrefined coconut oil
   (melted)

SUPPLIES

Pipette

Size 00 capsule (time-release capsules are preferred)

1. Using a pipette, drop the essential oils into the narrower, bottom half of the capsule.
2. Fill the remaining space in the capsule with the carrier oil of your choice.
3. Fit the wider, top half of the capsule over the bottom half and secure snugly.
4. Swallow the capsule immediately with water on an empty stomach.
5. Take once or twice daily for fourteen days.

Note: *Do not premake capsules and store for future use because you do not want them to leach or erode. This is just one of the many blends that you can use to treat inflammation orally and topically. Test different combinations of the oils listed above to see how your body responds, always consult with your health care provider to make sure no contraindications exist, and keep your topical dilutions to 2%–3%.*

ESSENTIAL OILS FOR SPECIFIC AUTOIMMUNE CONDITIONS

In spite of the limited research describing how essential oils interact with the root cause(s) of autoimmune disease, there are studies that discuss how they can potentially help manage common symptoms associated with a few specific conditions.

Ulcerative Colitis

A very promising 2007 animal study examined the anti-inflammatory effects of the combination of thyme and oregano essential oils at three dietary concentrations on mice with colitis.[21] The three concentrations they used were diluted in an edible carrier oil as follows:

1. 0.4% thyme and 0.2% oregano oils
2. 0.2% thyme and 0.1% oregano oils
3. 0.1% thyme and 0.05% oregano oils

It appeared that the medium dose did the trick, lowering a variety of pro-inflammatory cytokines and interleukins. Moreover, and this is the exciting part of this report: "Administration of the medium dose decreased the mortality rate, accelerated the body weight gain recovery, and reduced the macroscopic damage of the colonic tissue." In other words, the combination of 0.2% thyme and 0.1% oregano oils in an edible carrier can trigger a cascade of benefits like weight gain and can potentially expand life expectancy of animals with colitis!

But before you start to make your own diluted thyme and oregano capsules, remember that this is just one animal study and we still don't know how humans will respond to this mixture. Not to mention that treating ulcerative colitis in humans is a little trickier because the only way to ensure that essential oils will reach the colon is to take them internally via a time-release capsule—essential oils taken orally as a liquid solution or even in gel capsules will only be dissolved by gastric juices in the stomach. Also known as a "delayed-release" approach, enteric-coated capsules are designed to protect the stomach from gastric-irritating compounds and to dissolve only when they reach the intestines or colon.

In addition, if you are creating your own anti-inflammatory capsules under the guidance of your health care provider, keep in mind that essential oils rich in 1,8-cineole can be especially beneficial. According to a study published in the journal *Food and Chemical,* colitis-induced rats responded so well to the therapy that was devised that the researcher concluded, "These results confirm the anti-inflammatory action of 1,8-cineole and suggest its potential value as a dietary flavoring agent in the prevention of gastrointestinal inflammation and ulceration."[22]

Here is a list of oils you can easily purchase that contain a rich amount of 1,8-cineole:[23]

- Cajuput
- Cardamom
- *Eucalyptus globulus* and *radiata*
- Galangal
- Ho leaf
- Myrtle
- Niaouli
- Rosemary
- Sage
- Saro
- Spike lavender

To make your own capsules to fight colitis, remember that a little goes a long way, and always keep your health care provider in the loop, especially if you're currently taking immune-suppressing medications. Here are a couple different recipes to get you started.

COLITIS-SOOTHING CAPSULES

2 drops oregano essential oil
2 drops thyme essential oil
Organic, unrefined coconut oil or olive oil

SUPPLIES
Pipette
Size 00 time-release capsule

1. Using a pipette, drop the essential oils into the narrower, bottom half of the capsule.
2. Fill the remaining space in the capsule with coconut or olive oil.
3. Fit the wider, top half of the capsule over the bottom half and secure snugly.
4. Swallow a capsule immediately with water on an empty stomach. Take twice daily for up to four weeks.

Note: *Do not premake and store for future use.*

4 drops eucalyptus essential oil

3 drops rosemary essential oil

3 drops niaouli essential oil

3 drops galangal essential oil

Fractionated coconut oil or the carrier oil of your choice, as needed

SUPPLIES

10 ml glass roller bottle

1. Drop the essential oils into the roller bottle.

2. Fill the bottle with a carrier oil.

3. Massage over the abdomen, small of the back, and soles of the feet twice daily for two weeks.

Note: *As always, check the list of oils rich in 1,8-cineole on page 254 and, for any oils you don't own, substitute others that you may have on hand, like rosemary and even sage.*

Multiple Sclerosis

Affecting twice as many young women as men, multiple sclerosis (MS) usually settles in by the age of fifty. Aromatherapy techniques can be particularly effective at alleviating many nagging symptoms such as restlessness, sleep disturbance, joint and muscle rigidity, and not feeling well overall.[24] In my practice, I have seen MS patients get the best results when they use anti-inflammatory essential oils to alleviate pain and special blends to help improve mobility. Intentional movement therapies like tai chi, yoga, and even daily walks, are critical for MS patients, and few things can do as much as essential oils to soothe muscles and put someone into that meditative state of mind.

Application: Make the Movement Therapy Diffuser Blend and Roll-On below and make intentional motion part of your daily ritual.

MOVEMENT THERAPY DIFFUSER BLEND FOR MS

Yoga instructors often diffuse palo santo during their classes to help promote deep breathing and to inspire clear meditation.

2 drops palo santo essential oil
2 drops opoponax essential oil
2 drops bergamot essential oil

SUPPLIES
Diffuser

1. Drop the essential oils into the diffuser.
2. Fill with water to the indicated "fill line."
3. Using during intentional movement therapy sessions like tai chi, yoga, or walking to keep joints and muscles limber and loose.

MOVEMENT THERAPY ROLL-ON FOR MS

4 drops palo santo essential oil
3 drops bergamot essential oil
3 drops frankincense essential oil
3 drops myrrh essential oil
Fractionated coconut oil or the carrier oil of your choice

SUPPLIES
10 ml glass roller bottle

1. Drop the essential oils into the roller bottle.
2. Fill the remaining space in the bottle with a carrier oil.
3. Massage over joints and tight muscles minutes before movement therapy sessions like tai chi, yoga, or walking.

Rheumatoid Arthritis

One of the most promising studies on the use of essential oils to treat rheumatoid arthritis was published in 2005 by Korean researchers who evaluated how a special blend of essential oils helped arthritis patients. First they blended eucalyptus, lavender, marjoram, rosemary, and peppermint essential oils in proportions of 2:1:2:1:1. Then they created a 1.5% dilution by mixing these with a blend of almond oil (45%), apricot oil (45%), and jojoba oil (10%). Application of this solution on forty arthritic patients topically produced outstanding results. "Aromatherapy significantly decreased both the pain score and the depression score of the experimental group compared with the control group," the researchers stated, with no side effects reported![25]

When we are so focused on the actual pain, we sometimes forget about the side effects of pain like depression, anxiety, fear, and insomnia. How encouraging it is to see that essential oils may help with some of these symptoms!

Application: Find an anti-arthritis pain blend that works for you and mix up your protocol every other month.

ARTHRITIS PAIN-REDUCING OINTMENT

14 drops eucalyptus essential oil
14 drops sweet marjoram essential oil
7 drops lavender essential oil
7 drops peppermint essential oil
7 drops rosemary essential oil
2 ounces almond oil
2 ounces apricot oil
1 tablespoon jojoba oil

SUPPLIES
Medium glass bowl
Lotion dispenser or glass jar

1. Drop the essential oils into a bowl.
2. Add the almond, apricot, and jojoba oils and mix well.
3. Rub over sore, arthritic joints daily or as needed.
4. Store in a lotion dispenser or glass jar.

➡ To watch me make this Arthritis Pain-Reducing Ointment and to learn more about living a pain-free life, go to HealingPowerOfEssentialOils.com.

Additionally, turmeric essential oil (TEO) has been found to protect joints from inflammation in animal studies. Building on previous laboratory research that examined turmeric's anti-arthritic properties, researchers found that high oral doses of TEO—corresponding to 5,000 mg/d in humans—had anti-inflammatory effects specific to the joints. There may be a potential role for turmeric or its components in preventing or slowing rheumatic disease, but this has not yet been demonstrated.[26]

17

Perimenopause, Menopause, and Postmenopause

A woman must wait for her ovaries to die before she can get her rightful personality back. Postmenstrual is the same as premenstrual; I am once again what I was before the age of twelve: a female human being who knows that a month has thirty days, not twenty-five, and who can spend every one of them free of the shackles of that defect of body and mind known as femininity.

—FLORENCE KING

When I started to work with Mary, I learned that her perimenopause symptoms had lasted for more than a decade. Now in her midsixties, she suffered from osteopenia (low bone density), unexplained pain, insomnia, various gastrointestinal (GI) disorders, severe memory loss, emotional outbursts, fear, and bipolar disorder.

Due to the long-term litany of symptoms, I wanted her to experience some quick wins. We worked on some meal-planning strategies to cut out the main inflammatory triggers such as sugar, dairy, and gluten. Then we got her on a daily essential oil regimen to help her sleep better and to manage digestive upset and acid reflux. For insomnia I advised her to start diffusing my Sleepy-Time Blend (see page 50) about thirty minutes before bed. For stomach upset, constipation, and reflux I advised her to take one or two drops of my Healthy Digestion Blend (see page 50) in a gel capsule twice a day.

The first thing she noticed was near immediate relief of her GI complaints. Within days she was sleeping four to five hours a night—a marked improvement from the one-hour intermittent "naps" she was getting before. Only one hour at a time and then she'd wake up. Every. Single. Night.

Immediately, her energy levels skyrocketed and brain fog started to dissipate. Because she wasn't sleep deprived, she was able to manage her feelings better and wasn't always on an emotional roller coaster. We weren't able to fix everything on Mary's wish list, but she's made a lot of progress and she's been able to take up quilting again and do some other fun things with friends that she couldn't do before.

Every woman will go through a major life change when her body transforms from being fertile to infertile and her menstrual cycle stops. It is not a quick transition. It literally can last more than a decade, starting with perimenopause, evolving into menopause, and ending with the postmenopausal stage. If you asked the average woman what she knows about the "menopause experience," she would likely give you an answer relating to hot flashes and mood swings. It's no wonder, as our society and media have made these out to be the most prominent parts of this life change, and the butt of many jokes.

Interestingly, while menopause is a major life change that can bring uncomfortable symptoms, many women experience it as a freeing time. For those who no longer want to take birth control or manage natural family planning, menopause is also a welcomed event. It is no wonder that many women find themselves celebrating the end of a very long chapter of their lives where they had to deal with pads, tampons, and the inconvenience of the physical and emotional symptoms associated with the monthly cycle!

USING ESSENTIAL OILS FOR PERIMENOPAUSE

Perimenopause is defined as the period of time that starts with the onset of irregular menstrual cycles until your final menstrual period. It is marked by fluctuations in reproductive hormones that can cause a slew of undesirable effects.

For many women, perimenopausal symptoms are mild and do little to disrupt daily life. For others, life can get exceptionally challenging.[1] If you're in your late thirties or early forties and start to experience some of the following symptoms, you may be perimenopausal.

- Cholesterol imbalance
- Hot flashes
- Irregular periods
- Lowered libido
- Mood changes and irritability
- Sleep problems and fatigue

The good news is that you can manage your symptoms without the use of hormone replacement therapy and over-the-counter medications. For the growing number of women who wish to avoid prescription hormone medications, remedies like essential oils can provide natural and effective relief.

The only study I could find on treating perimenopause with essential oils suggests that essential oils have more of an ability to manage root cause hormonal imbalance than we initially anticipated. Thirty-one perimenopausal women applied 2.5 ml of cream (1.5% solution of vitex essential oil and a base oil or unscented lotion) on their skin once daily for five to seven days per week for a total of three months, and noticed a marked improvement in emotional problems and hot flashes.[2] The vitex solution also improved vaginal tone and lubrication, thereby facilitating a more pleasurable sexual experience, and helped moderate irregular periods. Because these symptoms are primarily caused by hormone disruption, the fact that vitex (an herb also known as chasteberry—see more information about vitex on page 267) helped these women reduce hot flashes and emotional disturbances suggests that it can play a key role in normalizing the imbalance in reproductive hormones that leads to these symptoms in the first place.

We have a long way to go in our understanding of how to best use essential oils for perimenopause as this area is still very much underresearched, but at least we have a good start! Experience has told me that you get the best results by taking a two-pronged approach: implementing an essential oils protocol designed to target both hormone balance and symptom relief. Like any condition, the key is to be proactive and to be aware of your body's changing environment.

I have personally observed that for many women, using a perimenopause balancing blend at the onset does the trick. If you can catch it in time, you'll be less likely to experience dramatic hormone fluctuations and, hopefully, coast through menopause with no problem at all.

PERIMENOPAUSE BALANCE BLEND

5 drops clary sage essential oil

5 drops geranium essential oil

5 drops lavender essential oil

5 drops vitex essential oil

5 drops ylang ylang essential oil

1 drop rose or jasmine absolute for an added floral touch (optional)

2 ounces evening primrose oil

SUPPLIES

Medium glass bowl

Lotion dispenser or glass jar

1. Drop the essential oils into the bowl.
2. Add the evening primrose oil and mix.
3. Massage over the abdomen at the onset of perimenopause symptoms twice a day for 3 to 4 weeks at a time. Switch to another blend every other month using menopause-friendly oils (see pages 264–268).
4. Store in a lotion dispenser or glass jar.

ESSENTIAL OILS FOR MENOPAUSE RELIEF

Typically experienced during your forties or fifties, menopause is traditionally defined as beginning twelve months after a woman's final menstrual period. It marks the official end of fertility and the menstrual cycle. When your body undergoes this change, estrogen levels begin to drop. As you can imagine, this fluctuation in hormone levels can cause a number of complaints that look very similar to perimenopause, although they are typically experienced much more intensely.

Unlike with perimenopause, we have much more research evaluating how essentials can be used to manage specific menopause symptoms. A 2008 article published in the *Evidence-Based Complementary and Alternative Medicine* journal summarizes what we know quite well: that many essential oils, including clary sage, fennel, cypress, angelica, and coriander, contain components that can act like estrogen in the body (the reduction of which can trigger many postmenopausal symptoms) and that evening primrose oil has benefits of its own when used as a carrier oil for these essential oils.[3] This article goes on to report how sixty menopausal women between the ages of forty-five and fifty-four responded to a series of essential oil massage treatments and measured the severity of these common menopausal symptoms:

- Arthralgia or myalgia (joint or muscle pain)
- Formication (sensation that insects are crawling on skin)
- Headache
- Hot flashes (vasomotor)
- Insomnia and sleep disturbances
- Nervousness
- Melancholia (deep sadness or gloom)
- Palpitations (rapid, strong, irregular heartbeat)
- Paresthesia (pins-and-needles feeling)
- Vertigo (loss of balance, sensation of whirling, dizziness)
- Weakness

Each participant received one thirty-minute aromatherapy treatment session per week for eight weeks with essential oils of lavender, rose geranium, rose, and jasmine diluted in almond and evening primrose oils. Compared to control subjects, the measured menopausal symptoms were greatly reduced in these women.

Whether one essential oil has more benefit over another still remains to be seen. At least we know this massage blend works!

SUPER MENOPAUSE MASSAGE BLEND

20 drops lavender essential oil

15 drops rose geranium essential oil

10 drops jasmine essential oil

5 drops rose absolute

2 ounces evening primrose oil

SUPPLIES

Medium glass bowl

Lotion dispenser or glass jar

1. Drop the essential oils into the bowl.
2. Add the evening primrose oil and mix.
3. Use as a full body massage oil or moisturizer twice a day for up to four weeks.
4. Be sure to switch to another blend every other month.
5. Store in a lotion dispenser or glass jar.

Following are five of the more promising essential oils for menopause and how to use them.

1. Clary Sage

Its floral notes, calming scent, and soothing attributes have made clary sage the go-to oil for women's health for centuries. Traditionally used to mitigate labor pain, it also offers antidepressant effects as described in a 2014 study that was conducted on twenty-two women in Korea.[4] The trial measured neurotransmitter levels found in blood samples of menopausal women and discovered that, by simply inhaling clary sage oil, levels of the stress hormone cortisol dropped considerably and serotonin levels were elevated. The result was an overall improvement in depression symptoms.

Application: Use in an inhaler (15-20 drops) or apply a 3% dilution of clary sage oil on the back of the neck or on the abdomen during bouts of depression.

Clary sage can also help with cramping. Yes, it is true that menopause signals the end of menstruation; however, during the beginning stages of menopause menstrual cramping can still occur. Try this cream to help prevent that from happening to you. If cramping persists or worsens during menopause, consult your health care provider immediately because this may be a sign of something more serious.

MENOPAUSE CRAMPING BODY CREAM

20 drops clary sage essential oil

15 drops lavender essential oil

10 drops ylang ylang essential oil

5 drops vitex essential oil

2 ounces unrefined shea butter

1 ounce evening primrose oil

1 ounce jojoba oil

SUPPLIES

Medium glass bowl

Lotion dispenser or glass jar

1. Drop the essential oils into a bowl.
2. Add the shea butter, evening primrose oil, and jojoba oil and mix.
3. Use as a body lotion two or three times per week.
4. Store in a lotion dispenser or glass jar.

2. Lavender

The shifting hormones of menopause can cause feelings of anxiety and problems with sleep. Lavender has long been known to promote feelings of relaxation while lifting mood, and for promoting better sleep in people dealing with insomnia.[5] Lavender aromatherapy will be a welcome addition to your nighttime routine during your change of life to help improve sleep and relaxation.

You can also use lavender to soothe menopause-related vaginal pain and soreness that can accompany vaginal dryness—something we don't hear too much about, but which can be quite irritating for women who are sexually active or who sit down a lot at work.

Application: Use a cold compress mixed with a 1% lavender oil dilution to reduce discomfort in the perineum during menopause.

PERINEUM COMPRESS

2 drops lavender essential oil
1 drop clary sage essential oil
1 tablespoon fractionated coconut oil
3 to 4 cups cold distilled water

SUPPLIES
Large glass bowl
Soft clean cloth

1. Mix the essential oils and fractionated coconut oil in the bowl.
2. Pour in the cold water. (You can also use warm water if desired.)
3. Soak the cloth in the solution, wring it out, and apply to the perineal area for a few moments to sooth soreness.
4. Soak the cloth again and repeat the process for 5 to 15 minutes.

3. Peppermint

Peppermint is a key essential oil to lessen discomfort during a hot flash and to give you a natural boost in energy. Misting your face with a water spritzer or using a portable inhaler during hot flash episodes or moments when you need pep in your step can have quick and dramatic results. Since hot flashes and fatigue are two of the most noticeable symptoms of menopause, having some peppermint oil on hand is a good idea.

Application: Create a spritzer by combining 10 drops of peppermint oil, 5 drops of witch hazel, and enough water to fill a 1-ounce spray bottle; use as needed.

4. Geranium

Geranium oil can help with many of the symptoms of menopause. It improves dry skin and is a popular ingredient in many women's blends for good reason. Like clary sage, in research geranium oil has been to shown to have antidepressant properties, so you can safely add it to your arsenal to manage mood swings and the blues.[6]

Application: Add 5 drops of geranium essential oil to the Menopause Cramping Body Cream (page 265) for added mood-boosting, antidepression support.

5. Vitex Agnus-Castus

An oil you may not be too familiar with, vitex agnus-castus (also known as chasteberry) essential oil is derived from a shrub that is native to Central Asia. It has blue-violet flowers; long, finger-shaped leaves; and dark purple berries; the fruit and seed are used to make medicine while the leaves and berries are distilled to make essential oils.

Vitex has been traditionally consumed for a variety of female health concerns, such as:

- Controlling bleeding
- Female infertility
- Helping the body force out the placenta after childbirth
- Increasing breast milk production
- "Lumpy" (fibrocystic) breasts
- Menopause
- Menstrual cycle irregularities
- Premenstrual dysphoric disorder (a more severe form of PMS)
- Premenstrual syndrome (PMS)
- Preventing miscarriage in women with low levels of progesterone

One study of vitex discovered that the essential oil extracted from the leaf appears to have a broader range of effective applications than the essential oil extracted from the berry, so try to get your hands on that type.[7]

Application: Put 3 drops vitex, 2 drops ylang ylang, and 1 drop Hawaiian sandalwood essential oil in your diffuser for a stabilizing aroma throughout the day.

MENOPAUSE RELIEF OINTMENT

This blend makes a great go-to body oil for menopause symptoms.

10 drops vitex essential oil

5 drops frankincense essential oil

5 drops Hawaiian sandalwood essential oil

5 drops ylang ylang essential oil

2 ounces evening primrose oil or Mama Z's Oil Base (page 43)

SUPPLIES

Medium glass bowl

Lotion dispenser or glass jar

1. Drop the essential oils into the bowl.
2. Add the evening primrose oil and mix.
3. Use as a massage oil or as part of your normal lotion rotation when symptoms are present.
4. Be sure to switch to another blend every other month.
5. Store in a lotion dispenser or glass jar.

MANAGING POSTMENOPAUSAL SYNDROME WITH ESSENTIAL OILS

Once menstruation has not occurred for twelve consecutive months, a woman is considered postmenopausal, meaning she is no longer fertile and her monthly "blessing" becomes a distant memory. Depending on how severely estrogen levels drop, it is common for women to find themselves experiencing a variety of conditions that make up what is known as "postmenopausal syndrome."[8]

- Cancer
- Cardiovascular disease
- Cognitive decline
- Osteoporosis
- Psychiatric symptoms
- Sexual problems
- Vasomotor symptoms like hot flashes or night sweats
- Urogenital atrophy

It can be difficult to distinguish between symptoms that result from loss of ovarian function and those that are due to aging. As a result, coming up with an accurate postmenopausal syndrome diagnosis can be problematic for health care providers. Be sure to talk to your provider if you are experiencing any of these symptoms of postmenopausal syndrome:[9]

- Depression
- Difficulty concentrating
- Dry vagina
- Headaches and migraines
- Insomnia
- Irritability
- Mental confusion
- Mood swings
- Osteoporotic symptoms
- Stress incontinence
- Urge incontinence
- Vasomotor symptoms like hot flashes or night sweats

The far-reaching effects of essential oils definitely don't stop at menopause, and many women find themselves using them well into their golden years. Since diagnosing postmenopausal syndrome can be so difficult, however, it's best to focus on condition-based management. Whether or not you have an official diagnosis of postmenopausal syndrome, you are likely to experience some of the same health conditions as you age.

Stress and Hypertension

Hypertension is often intricately linked to stress. A 2014 Korean study illustrates this point well.[10] Testing how sixty-three healthy postmenopausal women responded to inhaling 0.1% and 0.5% dilutions of neroli essential oil in an almond carrier, researchers uncovered some astounding findings. Compared to the control group, simply smelling neroli for five minutes two times a day for just five days had profound effects on their mind and body:

- Systolic blood pressure significantly lowered in the 0.5% neroli group only.
- Diastolic blood pressure significantly lowered in both the 0.1% and 0.5% neroli groups.

- Pulse rate and serum cortisol levels dropped in both groups, which indicates that stress was reduced.
- Estrogen concentrations and sex drive also improved in both groups.

Clearly, all of these factors do not work in isolation. Libido, hypertension, pulse rate, stress levels, and estrogen concentrations are all intricately linked. And to think that little ol' neroli can help all of that. Wow!

Want to experience the power? Try it for yourself!

Application: Make your own postmenopausal neroli inhaler and enjoy daily.

POSTMENOPAUSAL INHALER

15 to 20 drops neroli essential oil

SUPPLIES
Precut organic cotton pad
Aromatherapy inhaler

1. Place a cotton pad in the inhaler tube.
2. Drop the essential oil directly onto the cotton pad inside the tube.
3. Find a peaceful place in your house in the morning and enjoy a private neroli aromatherapy session before the day gets crazy. Sit down, relax, and gently breathe in the vapors from your inhaler for about five minutes.
4. Repeat before you go to bed.

Depression

Depression and menopause share many of the same symptoms, including anxiety, brain fog, fatigue, irritability, and sleep disturbances, just to name a few. Subsequently, many women suffer from undiagnosed (and untreated) depression during this stage of life. Unfortunately, this puts many at a disadvantage because it's far too easy to excuse or ignore these serious symptoms as being a rite of passage.

This is one reason why I'd like to see postmenopausal women using ylang

ylang on a regular basis. We've already seen how powerful this oil is for a variety of health conditions and for its harmonizing effects. Well, it's just as effective at helping women overcome depression! I can't say enough good things about ylang ylang. Antidepressive in nature with euphoric properties, it can help women suffering from low self-esteem and postmenopausal syndrome.[11]

Application: Make an inhaler similar to the recipe above but with ylang ylang, and enjoy!

Fat Burning

Who says that getting older is an excuse to see your body transform into something you can't stand looking at?

As I discussed back in chapter 8, research has found that massaging the abdomen (twice a day for six weeks) with a 3% solution of grapefruit and cypress oils helped women achieve significant decrease in abdominal fat and waist circumference.[12]

TUMMY TUCK SALVE

20 drops cypress essential oil
20 drops grapefruit essential oil
10 drops lime essential oil
10 drops peppermint essential oil
2 ounces unrefined shea butter
1 ounce jojoba oil

SUPPLIES
Medium glass bowl
Lotion dispenser or glass jar

1. Drop the essential oils into the bowl.
2. Add the shea butter and jojoba oil and mix.
3. Massage over the abdomen two or three times per week.
4. Store in a lotion dispenser or glass jar.

Vaginal Dryness and Atrophy

I get many requests from my Essential Oils Club members for oils to help with vaginal dryness and thinning of vaginal tissue. Estrogen helps the vagina remain lubricated with a thin layer of clear fluid, which helps keep the vaginal walls elastic, healthy, and thick. When your estrogen drops during menopause, this natural healing lubricant is reduced and your vaginal walls become thinner and less elastic. This is called vaginal atrophy and if vaginal dryness becomes bothersome, many doctors prescribe a topical estrogen cream.

I recommend avoiding all conventional store-bought douches, bubble baths, lotions, and scented soaps because the chemicals in these products can worsen dryness. Instead, consider making your own moisturizer and lubricant.

I am not aware of any essential oils that have been shown to "cure" vaginal dryness and vaginal atrophy, but I have been told by the women in my Essential Oils Club that they commonly enjoy a nice blend of highly diluted, gentle oils (0.5%–1%, or 3 to 6 drops of essential oils per ounce of carrier) as a lubricant before, during, and after sexual intercourse. Additionally, using the gentle vaginal lubricant (recipe follows) as a daily vaginal moisturizer can help reduce the friction that can occur when the labia rub together when walking and sitting.

GENTLE VAGINAL LUBRICANT

3 drops geranium essential oil

3 drops lavender essential oil

3 drops Roman chamomile essential oil

3 drops ylang ylang essential oil

2 ounces Mama Z's Oil Base (page 43) or straight jojoba oil—avoid coconut and fractionated coconut because they absorb too quickly

SUPPLIES

Medium glass bowl

Lotion dispenser or glass jar

1. Drop the essential oils into the bowl.

2. Add Mama Z's Oil Base and mix well. Store in a lotion dispenser or glass jar.

3. Massage into the labia before and after sexual intercourse and as needed. You may also find it helpful to lubricate your vagina after swimming and showering.

➡ To watch me and Mama Z make this Gentle Vaginal Lubricant and to learn more about managing vaginal dryness, go to HealingPowerOfEssentialOils.com.

Bone Loss

Changing hormone levels are a primary cause of osteoporosis, which can increase the risk of fractures.[13] This seems all but unavoidable to many women and an inevitable cause of permanent disability as they age. As such, postmenopausal women often take over-the-counter calcium supplements or prescription drugs to stave off bone density loss and osteoporosis.

There are three important things to keep in mind about bone density loss.

1. You can't avoid it, but you can slow it down. Considerably. Remember, *osteopenia* is simply the loss of bone density. *Osteoporosis* is a more serious condition that puts you at significant risk for fractures.

2. Regular weight-bearing exercise and a diet naturally rich in calcium (which includes dairy and leafy greens like spinach) are key.

3. Essential oils can help!

Essential oils of juniper, sage, rosemary, pine, dwarf pine, turpentine, and eucalyptus have been found to inhibit the breakdown and absorption of bone cells when added to food in animal studies. Pine oil, specifically, stood out as being able to protect from bone loss.[14]

BONE-STRENGTHENING CREAM

7 drops juniper essential oil

7 drops sage essential oil

7 drops rosemary essential oil

7 drops eucalyptus essential oil

7 drops pine essential oil

1 ounce unrefined shea butter

2 ounces Mama Z's Oil Base (page 43)

SUPPLIES

Medium glass bowl

Lotion dispenser or glass jar

1. Drop the essential oils into the bowl.
2. Add the shea butter and Mama Z's Oil Base and mix.
3. Apply as a moisturizer over your joints two or three times per week.
4. Store in a lotion dispenser or glass jar.

There are many ways to use natural therapies like essential oils to better enjoy your golden years. I think of Caleb in the Bible who, at eighty years old, wanted to go into battle to get the land that God had promised him. How many people do you know at eighty with that much energy and vigor?

Do you want to be one of them?

Then go! Get your Promised Land! It is your birthright to enjoy abundant life, health, and wellness well into your eighties, nineties, and hundreds!

Conclusion

And the leaves of the tree are for the healing of the nations.

REVELATION 22:2

After learning about all of the wonderful healing properties of essential oils, this verse has more meaning, doesn't it?

In this book, you have learned of the various ways essential oils can restore and bring balance to the mind, body, and spirit. They are truly God's gift to the world, and it all starts in nature. I hope that you will forever see each and every bark, flower, fruit, leaf, nut, resin, or root that you encounter through a new, more enlightened lens.

The healing power of essential oils can facilitate life transformation like few things on the planet, and it's important to remember that they should be used with care. Please don't forget the safety tips outlined in this book, and be sure to stick with the prescribed dilutions. The key to enjoying the health benefits of essential oils is to use them the right way, which will help ensure their effectiveness.

ONE LAST CHALLENGE

By definition, the chronic diseases that plague the world—such as cancer, diabetes, autoimmunity, and heart disease—take years to develop, so we should be armed with the reassurance that healing takes time. Never forget that there is no "quick fix." It just doesn't exist.

Healing is a process, and I invite you to join me on a personal journey to enjoying abundant life health, which means that we can never stop learning. Mastering the healing art and science of essential oils takes practice, and is a lifelong, trial-and-error experience.

The ancient Chinese philosopher and writer Lao Tzu once said, "The journey of a thousand miles begins with one step." Enjoy the journey, and know that there is always more to learn, and more healing available to you.

ACKNOWLEDGMENTS

My sincere love and heartfelt appreciation to God, and all of the behind-the-scenes people He put in my path who helped make this book happen.

To Miss Alex, Mama Z's right-hand gal and our children's nanny. Mary Poppins has got nothing on you, girl! Without your help, I cannot imagine how we would have survived this crazy season. We all love you!

To my right-hand gal online, Erica Mueller, you've been around since the very beginning. What a blessing you have been. I so value you as my Jacqueline-of-all-trades and, of course, my friend.

And to the rest of the DrEricZ.com team, your hard work and determination have been priceless! Thank you so much for all that you do to make DrEricZ.com the number one most-visited website devoted to biblical health on the planet!

To Sylla Sheppard-Hanger, CMT, founder of the Atlantic Institute of Aromatherapy, and my fellow aromatherapy colleagues for peer-reviewing this manuscript to ensure that it is not only factually accurate but also honors the art and science of aromatherapy: Lauren Bridges, AMP; Ken Miller, AMP; Hui Ling; and Janet Roark, DVM.

To my literary agent, John Maas, and the team at Sterling Lord Literistic, for your advocacy, hard work, and for being my trusted guide. You are the best!

To my editor and right-hand gal, Kate Hanley, for your brilliant insight and savvy wordsmithing. Yay, we did it!

To the wonderful team at Harmony Books: Alyse Diamond, Christina Foxley, Maya Lane, Michele Eniclerico, Tammy Blake, Estefania Ospina, and the unsung heroes in the fact-checking and copyediting departments—all I can say is, "Wow!"

You are the dream team and an author couldn't have asked for a better group of professionals to make all of this happen.

Last, but not least, to all of my Inner Circle members, newsletter subscribers, and social media followers, for your thought-provoking questions, kind comments, and unending support. You are the reason I do what I do, and I thank you for helping spread this message to millions of people across the globe!

NOTES

Introduction

1. World Health Organization, "Constitution of WHO: Principles," http://www.who.int/about/mission/en, accessed April 5, 2017.
2. T. F. Hodge, *From Within I Rise* (Baltimore: PublishAmerica, 2009), 44.

Part 1: ESSENTIAL OILS REVOLUTION

1. L. Stokowski, "Can We Stop Overprescribing Antibiotics? Readers Speak Out," Medscape, http://www.medscape.com/viewarticle/827888, accessed April 4, 2017.

Chapter 1: FUNDAMENTALS OF AROMATHERAPY

1. *Encyclopaedia Brittanica*, s.v. "Essential Oils," https://www.britannica.com/topic/essential-oil.
2. Ibid.
3. B. Saad and O. Said, *Greco-Arab and Islamic Herbal Medicine* (Malden, Mass.: John Wiley & Sons, 2011).
4. Ibid.
5. J. Buckle, *Clinical Aromatherapy,* 3rd edition (London: Churchill Livingstone, 2014), 9–10.
6. Free Dictionary, s.v. "Fixed Oil," http://medical-dictionary.thefreedictionary.com/fixed+oil.
7. *Encyclopaedia Brittanica*, "Essential Oils."
8. S. Price and L. Price, *Aromatherapy for Health Professionals,* 4th edition (London: Churchill Livingstone, 2011), 5.
9. G. K. Jayaprakasha and L. J. M. Rao, "Chemistry, Biogenesis, and Biological Activities of *Cinnamomum zeylanicum*," *Critical Reviews in Food Science and Nutrition* 51, no. 6 (2011): 547–562. DOI: 10.1080/10408391003699550.
10. Price and Price, *Aromatherapy for Health Professionals,* 6.
11. Atlantic Institute of Aromatherapy, *Aromatherapy Practitioner Course* (Tampa, Fla.: Atlantic Institute of Aromatherapy), 61.
12. Price and Price, *Aromatherapy for Health Professionals,* 10–11.
13. N. Zouari, "Essential Oils Chemotypes: A Less Known Side," *Medicinal and Aromatic Plants* 2 (2013). DOI:10.4172/2167-0412.1000e145.
14. Interview with Robert Pappas, "Debunking the Most Common (and Dangerous!) Myths," Essential Oils Revolution 2 Online Summit, August 2016.
15. Interview with Robert Pappas, "Essential Oil Preparation," Essential Oils Revolution Online Summit, May 2015.
16. D. W. Light, J. Lexchin, and J. J. Darrow, "Institutional Corruption of Pharmaceuticals and the Myth of Safe and Effective Drugs," *Journal of Law, Medicine and Ethics* 14, no. 3 (2013): 590–610.
17. J. B. Mowry et al., "2013 Annual Report of the American Association of Poison Control Centers' National Poison Data System (NPDS): 31st Annual Report," *Clinical Toxicology* 52 (2014): 1032–1283. DOI: 10.3109/15563650.2.
18. Ibid.
19. The National Center for Biotechnology Information, https://www.ncbi.nlm.nih.gov/pubmed/?term=menthol, accessed April 8, 2017.
20. The National Center for Biotechnology Information,

https://www.ncbi.nlm.nih.gov/pubmed/?term=pep permint+essential+oil, accessed April 8, 2017.

21. A. Borhani Haghighi et al., "Cutaneous Application of Menthol 10% Solution as an Abortive Treatment of Migraine Without Aura: A Randomised, Double-blind, Placebo-controlled, Crossed-over Study," *International Journal of Clinical Practice* 64 (2010): 451–456. DOI: 10.1111/j.1742–1241.2009.02215.x.

22. M. Tognolini, "Protective Effect of Foeniculum vulgare Essential Oil and Anethole in an Experimental Model of Thrombosis," *Pharmacological Research* 56, no. 3 (2007): 254–260. DOI: 10.1016/j .phrs.2007.07.002.

23. L. Gori et al., "Can Estragole in Fennel Seed Decoctions Really Be Considered a Danger for Human Health? A Fennel Safety Update," *Evidence-Based Complementary and Alternative Medicine* (2012): DOI:10.1155/2012/860542.

24. E. C. Miller, "Structure-activity Studies of the Carcinogenicities in the Mouse and Rat of Some Naturally Occurring and Synthetic Alkenylbenzene Derivatives Related to Safrole and Estragole," *Cancer Research* 43, no. 3 (1983): 1124–1134.

25. L. Gori et al., "Can Estragole in Fennel Seed Decoctions Really Be Considered a Danger for Human Health? A Fennel Safety Update," *Evidence-Based Complementary and Alternative Medicine*, ID no. 860542 (2012). DOI: 10.1155/2012/860542.

26. L. Harris, "Essential Oils and Cancer—Potentially Carcinogenic and Anticarcinogenic Essential Oils," Using Essential Oils Safely, http://www.usingeos safely.com/essential-oils-and-cancer-potentially -carcinogenic-and-anti-carcinogenic-essential -oils, accessed April 8, 2017; "Cancer, Carcinogenesis and Essential Oils in Aromatherapy," Esoteric Oils, http://essentialoils.co.za/cancer.htm, accessed 4/8/17.

Chapter 2: BASIC TOOLS AND TECHNIQUES

1. Research conducted by Robert Pappas and reported on his Facebook page, April 6, 2017, https://www .facebook.com/EODoctor/posts/18226856546 63807.

2. D. Petersen, "An Aromatherapist's Report from IFEAT 2014: Pesticides, Cultured Aromas, the Arab Spring, and Global Warming," American College of Healthcare Sciences, http://info.achs.edu/ blog/an-aromatherapist-s-report-from-ifeat-2014 -pesticides-cultured-aromas-the-arab-spring-and -global-warming, accessed April 10, 2017.

3. Agency for Toxic Substances and Disease Registry, "Public Health Statement for Propylene Glycol," https://www.atsdr.cdc.gov/phs/phs.asp?id=1120 &tid=240, accessed April 10, 2017.

4. A. J. Mehta et al., "Heart Rate Variability in Association with Frequent Use of Household Sprays and Scented Products in SAPALDIA," *Environmental Health Perspectives* 120, no. 7 (2012): 958–964. DOI: 10.1289/ehp.1104567; A. Steinemann, "Ten Questions Concerning Air Fresheners and Indoor Built Environments," *Building and Environment* 111 (2017): 279–284. DOI: 10.1016/j.build env.2016.11.009.

5. I. Singh and A. P Morris, "Performance of Transdermal Therapeutic Systems: Effects of Biological Factors," *International Journal of Pharmaceutical Investigation* 1, no. 1 (2011): 4–9. DOI: 10.4103/2230 -973X.76721.

6. R. Tisserand and R. Young, *Essential Oil Safety: A Guide for Health Care Professionals*, 2nd ed. London: Churchill Livingstone, 2013), 85–87.

7. National Association for Holistic Aromatherapy, "Safety Information," http://naha.org/?/explore -aromatherapy/safety, accessed April 10, 2017.

8. Tisserand and Young, *Essential Oil Safety*.

9. S. Skalli and R. Soulaymani Bencheikh, "Epileptic Seizure Induced by Fennel Essential Oil," *Epileptic Disorders* 13, no. 3 (2011): 345–347. DOI:10.1684/ epd.2011.0451.

Chapter 3: STOCKING YOUR MEDICINE CABINET

1. K. M. Adams, W. S. Butsch, and M. Kohlmeier, "The State of Nutrition Education at US Medical Schools," *Journal of Biomedical Education* 2015, no. 357627 (2015). DOI:10.1155/2015/357627.

2. Ibid.

3. D. Wang et al., "Neuroprotective Activity of Lav-

ender Oil on Transient Focal Cerebral Ischemia in Mice," *Molecules* 17 (2012): 9803–9817. DOI: 10.3390/molecules17089803.

4. M. Hancianu et al., "Neuroprotective Effects of Inhaled Lavender Oil on Scopolamine-induced Dementia via Anti-oxidative Activities in Rats," *Phytomedicine* 20, no. 5 (2013): 446–452. DOI: 10.1016/j.phymed.2012.12.005.

5. H. Sebai et al., "Lavender (*Lavandula stoechas L.*) Essential Oils Attenuate Hyperglycemia and Protect Against Oxidative Stress in Alloxan-Induced Diabetic Rats," *Lipids in Health and Disease* 12, no. 1 (2013): 189.

6. S. Kasper, "An Orally Administered Lavandula Oil Preparation (Silexan) for Anxiety Disorder and Related Conditions: An Evidence Based Review," *International Journal of Psychiatry in Clinical Practice* 17, Suppl. 1 (2013): 15–22. DOI: 0.3109/13651501.2013.813555.

7. S. De Rapper et al., "The *In Vitro* Antimicrobial Activity of *Lavandula angustifolia* Essential Oil in Combination with Other Aroma-Therapeutic Oils," *Evidence-Based Complementary and Alternative Medicine* 2013, ID no. 852049 (2013). DOI: 10.1155/2013/852049.

8. D. T. Altaei, "Topical Lavender Oil for the Treatment of Recurrent Aphthous Ulceration," *American Journal of Dentistry* 25, no. 1 (2012): 39–43; H.-M. Kim and S.-H. Cho, "Lavender Oil Inhibits Immediate-type Allergic Reaction in Mice and Rats," *Journal of Pharmacy and Pharmacology* 51 (1999): 221–226. DOI: 10.1211/0022357991772178.

9. R. Tisserand and R. Young, *Essential Oil Safety: A Guide for Health Care Professionals*, 2nd ed. (London: Churchill Livingstone, 2013), 327.

10. D. V. Henley et al., "Prepubertal Gynecomastia Linked to Lavender and Tea Tree Oils," *New England Journal of Medicine* 356 (2007): 479–485. DOI: 10.1056/NEJMoa064725.

11. R. Tisserand, "Lavender Oil Is Not Carcinogenic," http://roberttisserand.com/2013/02/lavender-oil-is-not-estrogenic/, accessed April 9, 2017.

12. V. T. Politano et al., "Uterotrophic Assay of Percutaneous Lavender Oil in Immature Female Rats," *International Journal of Toxicology* 32, no. 2 (2013). DOI: 10.1177/1091581812472209.

13. P. S. X. Yap et al., "Combination of Essential Oils and Antibiotics Reduce Antibiotic Resistance in Plasmid-conferred Multidrug Resistant Bacteria," *Phytomedicine* 20, nos. 8–9 (2013): 710–713. DOI: 10.1016/j.phymed.2013.02.013.

14. M. F. Maia and S. J. Moore, "Plant-Based Insect Repellents: A Review of Their Efficacy, Development and Testing," *Malaria Journal*, 10, suppl. 1 (2011): S11. DOI: 10.1186/1475-2875-10-S1-S11.

15. Tisserand and Young, *Essential Oil Safety*, 387.

16. R. Nesmith, "Can Peppermint and Eucalyptus Be Used on Young Children?," *Essential Oils Blog*, Plant Therapy, January 29, 2014, https://www.planttherapy.com/blog/2014/01/29/can-peppermint-and-eucalyptus-be-used-on-young-children/, accessed April 9, 2017.

17. S. Sugumar et al., "Ultrasonic Emulsification of Eucalyptus Oil Nanoemulsion: Antibacterial Activity Against Staphylococcus Aureus and Wound Healing Activity in Wistar Rats," *Ultrasonics Sonochemistry* 21, no. 3 (2014): 1044–1049. DOI: 10.1016/j.ultsonch.2013.10.021.

18. Tisserand and Young, *Essential Oil Safety*, 273.

19. Nesmith, "Can Peppermint and Eucalyptus Be Used on Young Children?"

20. D. Hamdan, "Chemical Composition of the Essential Oils of Variegated Pink-fleshed Lemon (Citrus x limon L. Burm. f.) and Their Anti-inflammatory and Antimicrobial Activities," *Zeitschrift fur Naturforschung C: A Journal for Biosciences* 68, nos. 7–8 (2013): 275–284.

21. Y. Ozogul et al., "Antimicrobial Impacts of Essential Oils on Food Borne-Pathogens," *Recent Patents on Food, Nutrition and Agriculture* 7, no. 1 (2015): 53–61. DOI: 0.2174/2212798407666150615112153.

22. Tisserand and Young, *Essential Oil Safety*, 327.

23. A. Al-Harras et al., "Analgesic Effects of Crude Extracts and Fractions of Omani Frankincense Obtained from Traditional Medicinal Plant *Boswellia sacra* on Animal Models," *Asian Pacific Journal of Tropical Medicine* 7, no. 1 (2014): S485–S490. DOI: 10.1016/S1995-7645(14)60279-0.

24. E. J. Blain, A. Y. Ali, and V. C. Duance, "*Boswellia frereana* (Frankincense) Suppresses Cytokine-induced Matrix Metalloproteinase Expression and Production of Pro-inflammatory Molecules in Articular Cartilage," *Phytotherapy Research* 24 (2010): 905–912. DOI:10.1002/ptr.3055.

25. Y. Chen et al., "Composition and Potential Anticancer Activities of Essential Oils Obtained from Myrrh and Frankincense," *Oncology Letters* 6 (2013): 1140–1146. DOI: 10.3892/ol.2013.1520.

26. M. B. Frank et al., "Frankincense Oil Derived from *Boswellia carteri* Induces Tumor Cell Specific Cytotoxicity," *BMC Complementary and Alternative Medicine* 9, no. 6 (2009). DOI: 10.1186/1472-6882-9-6.

27. K. M. Fung et al., "Management of Basal Cell Carcinoma of the Skin Using Frankincense (*Boswellia sacra*) Essential Oil: A Case Report," *OA Alternative Medicine* 1, no. 2 (2013): 14.

28. Tisserand and Young, *Essential Oil Safety,* 327.

29. L. F. Fernandez, O. M. Palomino, and G. Frutos, "Effectiveness of *Rosmarinus officinalis* Essential Oil as Antihypotensive Agent in Primary Hypotensive Patients and Its Influence on Health-related Quality of Life," *Journal of Ethnopharmacology* 151, no. 1 (2014): 509–516. DOI: 10.1016/j.jep.2013.11.006.

30. W. Wang, "Antibacterial Activity and Anticancer Activity of *Rosmarinus officinalis* L. Essential Oil Compared to That of Its Main Components," *Molecules 17*, no. 3, (2012): 2704–2713. DOI:10.3390/molecules17032704.

31. Tisserand and Young, *Essential Oil Safety,* 409.

32. Ibid., 441.

33. L. T. H. Tan et al., "Traditional Uses, Phytochemistry, and Bioactivities of *Cananga odorata* (Ylang-Ylang)," *Evidence-Based Complementary and Alternative Medicine* 2015, ID no. 896314 (2015): 30 pages. DOI: 10.1155/2015/896314.

34. T. Hongratanaworakit and G. Buchbauer, "Evaluation of the Harmonizing Effect of Ylang-Ylang Oil on Humans After Inhalation," *Planta Medica* 70, no. 7 (2004): 632–636.

35. Tisserand and Young, *Essential Oil Safety,* 478.

36. P. Anitha and M. Indira, "Impact of Feeding Etha-nolic Extract of Root Bark of *Cananga odorata* (Lam) on Reproductive Functions in Male Rats," *Indian Journal of Experimental Biology* 44, no. 12 (2006): 976–980.

Chapter 4: QUICK-START GUIDE TO USING ESSENTIAL OILS TO CHANGE YOUR LIFE

1. W. Jager et al., "Percutaneous Absorption of Lavender Oil from a Massage Oil," *Journal of the Society of Cosmetic Chemists* 43, no. 1 (1992): 49–54.

2. M. Hardy et al., "Replacement of Drug Treatment for Insomnia by Ambient Odour," *Lancet* 346, no. 8976 (1995): 701.

3. K. M. Chang and C. W. Shen, "Aromatherapy Benefits Autonomic Nervous System Regulation for Elementary School Faculty in Taiwan," *Evidence-Based Complementary and Alternative Medicine* 2011, ID no. 946537 (2011): DOI: 10.1155/2011/946537.

4. C. Deng, "Aromatherapy: Exploring Olfaction," *Yale Scientific* 21 (2011): 25.

5. Y. Wu et al., "The Metabolic Responses to Aerial Diffusion of Essential Oils," *PLoS ONE* 7, no. 9 (2012): e44830. DOI:10.1371/journal.pone.0044830; J. K. Kiecolt-Glaser et al., "Olfactory Influences on Mood and Autonomic, Endocrine, and Immune Function," *Psychoneuroendocrinology* 33, no. 3 (2008): 328–339. DOI:10.1016/j.psyneuen.2007.11.015.

6. T. Friedman, "Attention Deficit and Hyperactivity Disorder (ADHD)," http://files.meetup.com/1481956/ADHD%20Research%20by%20Dr.%20Terry%20Friedmann.pdf, accessed April 7, 2017.

7. D. Jimbo, "Effect of Aromatherapy on Patients with Alzheimer's Disease," *Psychogeriatrics* 9, no. 4 (2009): 173–179. DOI: 10.1111/j.1479-8301.2009.00299.x.

8. M.-H. Hur et al. "Aromatherapy Massage on the Abdomen for Alleviating Menstrual Pain in High School Girls: A Preliminary Controlled Clinical Study," *Evidence-Based Complementary and Alternative Medicine* 2012, ID no. 187163 (2012). DOI: 10.1155/2012/187163.

9. M.-C. Ou et al., "Pain Relief Assessment by Aromatic Essential Oil Massage on Outpatients with Primary Dysmenorrhea: A Randomized, Double-blind Clinical Trial," *Journal of Obstetrics and Gyn-

aecology Research 38 (2012): 817–822. DOI: 10.1111/j.1447-0756.2011.01802.x.

10. K.-B. Lee, E. Cho, and Y. S. Kang, "Changes in 5-hydroxytryptamine and Cortisol Plasma Levels in Menopausal Women After Inhalation of Clary Sage Oil," *Phytotherapy Research* 28 (2014): 1599–1605. DOI: 10.1002/ptr.5163.

11. S. Y. Choi et al., "Effects of Inhalation of Essential Oil of *Citrus aurantium* L. var. *amara* on Menopausal Symptoms, Stress, and Estrogen in Postmenopausal Women: A Randomized Controlled Trial," *Evidence-Based Complementary and Alternative Medicine* 2014, ID no. 796518 (2014). DOI: 10.1155/2014/796518.

12. K. Nagai et al., "Olfactory Stimulatory with Grapefruit and Lavender Oils Change Autonomic Nerve Activity and Physiological Function," *Autonomic Neuroscience: Basic and Clinical* 185 (2014): 29–35. DOI: 10.1016/j.autneu.2014.06.005.

13. M. Hyman, "How to Stop Attacking Yourself: 9 Steps to Heal Autoimmune Disease," http://drhyman.com/blog/2010/07/30/how-to-stop-attacking-yourself-9-steps-to-heal-autoimmune-disease/, accessed March 27, 2017.

14. U.S. National Library of Medicine, "What Is an Inflammation?," https://www.ncbi.nlm.nih.gov/pubmedhealth/PMH0072482/, accessed March 27, 2017.

15. A. G. Guimarães, J. S. S. Quintans, and L. J. Quintans-Júnior, "Monoterpenes with Analgesic Activity—A Systematic Review," *Phytotherapy Research* 27 (2013): 1–15. DOI: 10.1002/ptr.4686.

Chapter 5: GETTING STARTED

1. P. Lally et al., "How Are Habits Formed: Modelling Habit Formation in the Real World," *European Journal of Social Psychology* 40 (2010): 998–1009. DOI:10.1002/ejsp.674.

2. Ibid.

Chapter 6: EXPANDING YOUR MEDICINE CABINET

1. D. Lo Furno et al., "A Citrus bergamia Extract Decreases Adipogenesis and Increases Lipolysis by Modulating PPAR Levels in Mesenchymal Stem Cells from Human Adipose Tissue," *PPAR Research* 2016, no. 4563815 (2016). DOI: 10.1155/2016/4563815.

2. E. Watanabe et al., "Effects of Bergamot (*Citrus bergamia* [Risso] Wright & Arn.) Essential Oil Aromatherapy on Mood States, Parasympathetic Nervous System Activity, and Salivary Cortisol Levels in 41 Healthy Females," *Forschende Komplementarmedizin* 22 (2015): 43–49. DOI: 10.1159/000380989.

3. K. Fisher and C. A. Phillips, "The Effect of Lemon, Orange and Bergamot Essential Oils and Their Components on the Survival of *Campylobacter jejuni, Escherichia coli* O157, *Listeria monocytogenes, Bacillus cereus* and *Staphylococcus aureus in vitro* and in Food Systems," *Journal of Applied Microbiology* 101 (2006): 1232–1240. DOI: 10.1111/j.1365-2672.2006.03035.x.

4. C.-H. Ni et al., "The Anxiolytic Effect of Aromatherapy on Patients Awaiting Ambulatory Surgery: A Randomized Controlled Trial," *Evidence-Based Complementary and Alternative Medicine* 2013, ID no. 927419 (2013). DOI: 10.1155/2013/927419.

5. K. Dimas et al., "The Effect of Sclareol on Growth and Cell Cycle Progression of Human Leukemic Cell Lines," *Leukemia Research* 23, no. 3 (1999): 217–234; L. Wang et al., "Sclareol, a Plant Diterpene, Exhibits Potent Antiproliferative Effects via the Induction of Apoptosis and Mitochondrial Membrane Potential Loss in Osteosarcoma Cancer Cells," *Molecular Medicine Reports* 11, no. 6 (2015): 4273. DOI: 10.3892/mmr.2015.3325.

6. C. M. Marya et al., "*In Vitro* Inhibitory Effect of Clove Essential Oil and Its Two Active Principles on Tooth Decalcification by Apple Juice," *International Journal of Dentistry* 759618 (2012). DOI: 10.1155/2012/759618.

7. I. Alexandrovich, "The Effect of Fennel (*Foeniculum vulgare*) Seed Oil Emulsion in Infantile Colic: A Randomized, Placebo-controlled Study," *Alternative Therapies in Health and Medicine* 9, no. 4 (2003): 58–61.

8. M. N. Boukhatem et al., "Rose Geranium Essential Oil as a Source of New and Safe Anti-inflammatory Drugs," *Libyan Journal of Medicine* 8 (2013). DOI:

10.3402/ljm.v8i0.22520; S. Pattnaik, V. R. Subramanyam, and C. Kole, "Antibacterial and Antifungal Activity of Ten Essential Oils in Vitro," *Microbios* 86, no. 349 (1996): 237–246.

9. M. A. Saleh, S. Clark, B. Woodard, and S. A. Deolu-Sobogun, "Antioxidant and Free Radical Scavenging Activities of Essential Oils," *Ethnicity and Disease* 20, no. 1, Suppl 1. (2010): S1–78–82.

10. R. M. Queiroz, "Apoptosis-inducing Effects of *Melissa officinalis L.* Essential Oil in Glioblastoma Multiforme Cells," *Cancer Investigations* 32, no. 6 (2014): 226–235. DOI: 10.3109/07357907.2014.905587.

11. M. Chung et al., "Anti-diabetic Effects of Lemon Balm (*Melissa officinalis*) Essential Oil on Glucose- and Lipid-regulating Enzymes in Type 2 Diabetic Mice," *British Journal of Nutrition* 104, no. 2 (2010): 180–188. DOI: 10.1017/S0007114510001765.

12. G. Shah et al., "Scientific Basis for the Therapeutic Use of *Cymbopogon citratus,* Stapf (Lemon grass)," *Journal of Advanced Pharmaceutical Technology & Research* 2, no. 1 (2011): 3–8. DOI: 10.4103/2231 -4040.79796.

13. Y. Chen et al., "Composition and Potential Anticancer Activities of Essential Oils Obtained from Myrrh and Frankincense," *Oncology Letters* 6, no. 4 (2013): 1140–1146. DOI: 10.3892/ol.2013.1520.

14. Ibid.

15. P. Khodabakhsh, H. Shafaroodi, and J. Asgarpanah, "Analgesic and Anti-inflammatory Activities of *Citrus aurantium* L. Blossoms Essential Oil (Neroli): Involvement of the Nitric Oxide/Cyclic-Guanosine Monophosphate Pathway," *Journal of Natural Medicine* 69, no. 3 (2015): 324–331. DOI:10.1007/s11418 -015-0896-6.

16. I.-H. Kim et al., "Essential Oil Inhalation on Blood Pressure and Salivary Cortisol Levels in Prehypertensive and Hypertensive Subjects," *Evidence-Based Complementary and Alternative Medicine* 2012, ID no. 984203 (2012). DOI: 10.1155/2012/984203.

17. T. Azanchi, H. Shafaroodi, and J. Asgarpanah, "Anticonvulsant Activity of *Citrus aurantium* Blossom Essential Oil (Neroli): Involvement of the GABAergic System," *Natural Product Communications* 9, no. 11 (2014): 1615–1618.

18. A. Bommareddy et al., "α-Santalol, a Derivative of Sandalwood Oil, Induces Apoptosis in Human Prostate Cancer Cells by Causing Caspase-3 Activation," *Phytomedicine* 19, nos. 8–9 (2012): 804–811. DOI: 10.1016/j.phymed.2012.04.003; S. Santha and C. Dwivedi, "Anticancer Effects of Sandalwood (*Santalum album*)," *Anticancer Research* 35, no. 6 (2015): 3137–3145; G. Kyle, "Evaluating the Effectiveness of Aromatherapy in Reducing Levels of Anxiety in Palliative Care Patients: Results of a Pilot Study," *Complementary Therapies in Clinical Practice* 12, no. 2 (2006): 148–155.

19. T. Hongratanaworakit, E. Heuberger, and G. Buchbauer, "Evaluation of the Effects of East Indian Sandalwood Oil and α-Santalol on Humans after Transdermal Absorption," *Planta Medica* 70, no. 1 (2004): 3–7. DOI: 10.1055/s-2004-815446; S. Y. Choi and K. Park, "Effect of Inhalation of Aromatherapy Oil on Patients with Perennial Allergic Rhinitis: A Randomized Controlled Trial," *Evidence-Based Complementary and Alternative Medicine* 2016, ID no. 7896081 (2016). DOI: 10.1155/2016 /7896081.

20. T. Friedmann, "Attention Deficit and Hyperactivity Disorder (ADHD)," http://files.meetup.com /1481956/ADHD%20Research%20by%20Dr.%20 Terry%20Friedmann.pdf, accessed April 10, 2017.

21. R. N. Campos, "Acaricidal Properties of Vetiver Essential Oil from *Chrysopogon zizanioides* (Poaceae) Against the Tick Species *Amblyomma cajennense* and *Rhipicephalus (Boophilus) Microplus* (Acari: Ixodidae)," *Veterinary Parasitology* 15, no. 212 (2015): 324–330. DOI: 10.1016/j.vetpar.2015.08.022.

22. T. Shen and H.-X. Lou, "Bioactive Constituents of Myrrh and Frankincense, Two Simultaneously Prescribed Gum Resins in Chinese Traditional Medicine," *Chemistry & Biodiversity* 5 (2008): 540–553. DOI: 10.1002/cbdv.200890051.

23. S. Cassella, J. P. Cassella, and I. Smith, "Synergistic Antifungal Activity of Tea Tree (*Melaleuca alternifolia*) and Lavender (*Lavandula angustifolia*) Essential Oils Against Dermatophyte Infection," *International Journal of Aromatherapy* 12, no. 1 (2002): 2–15. DOI: 10.1054/ijar.2001.0127.

24. M. Navarra et al., "*Citrus bergamia* Essential Oil: From Basic Research to Clinical Application," *Frontiers in Pharmacology* 6, no. 36 (2015). DOI: 10.3389/fphar.2015.00036.

25. National Center for Biotechnology Information, "(+) Limonene," https://pubchem.ncbi.nlm.nih.gov/compound/440917, accessed April 12, 2017.

26. H. Xiao et al., "Monodemethylated Polymethoxyflavones from Sweet Orange (*Citrus sinensis*) Peel Inhibit Growth of Human Lung Cancer Cells by Apoptosis," *Molecular Nutrition Food Research* 53, no. 3: 398–406. DOI: 10.1002/mnfr.200800057.

27. D. Jimbo et al., "Effect of Aromatherapy on Patients with Alzheimer's Disease," *Psychogeriatrics* 9, no. 4 (2009): 173–179. DOI: 10.1111/j.1479-8301.2009.00299.x.

28. J. Lehrner, "Ambient Odors of Orange and Lavender Reduce Anxiety and Improve Mood in a Dental Office," *Physiology & Behavior* 86, nos. 1–2 (2005): 92–95. DOI: 10.1016/j.physbeh.2005.06.031.

29. Y. B. Yip et al., "An Experimental Study on the Effectiveness of Massage with Aromatic Ginger and Orange Essential Oil for Moderate-to-Severe Knee Pain Among the Elderly in Hong Kong," *Complementary Therapies in Medicine* 16, no. 3 (2008): 131–138. DOI: 10.1016/j.ctim.2007.12.003.

30. S. Pattnaik, V. R. Subramanyam, and C. Kole, "Antibacterial and Antifungal Activity of Ten Essential Oils in Vitro," *Microbios* 866, no. 349 (1996): 237–246.

31. J. Sun, "D-Limonene: Safety and Clinical Applications," *Alternative Medicine Review* 12, no. 3 (2007): 259–264.

32. National Toxicology Program, National Toxicology Program Technical Report Series, "NTP Toxicology and Carcinogenesis Studies of d-Limonene (CAS No. 5989-27-5) in F344/N Rats and B6C3F1 Mice (Gavage Studies)," https://ntp.niehs.nih.gov/go/10574, accessed April 12, 2017.

33. H. Igimi, T. Hisatsugu, and M. Nishimura, "The Use of d-Limonene Preparation as a Dissolving Agent of Gallstones," *American Journal of Digestive Diseases* 21, no. 11 (1976): 926–939.

34. J. Sun, "D-Limonene: Safety and Clinical Applications," *Alternative Medicine Review* 12, no. 3 (2007): 259–264.

35. Ibid.

36. B. Mizrahi, "Citrus Oil and MgCl2 as Antibacterial and Anti-Inflammatory Agents," *Journal of Periodontology* 77, no. 6 (2006): 963–968. DOI: 10.1902/jop.2006.050278; W.-J. Yoon, N. H. Lee, and C.-G. Hyun, "Limonene Suppresses Lipopolysaccharide-Induced Production of Nitric Oxide, Prostaglandin E2, and Pro-inflammatory Cytokines in RAW 264.7 Macrophages," *Journal of Oleo Science* 59, no. 8 (2010): 415–421. DOI: 10.5650/jos.59.415.

37. V. A. Santiago et al., "Dietary d-Limonene Alleviates Insulin Resistance and Oxidative Stress–induced Liver Injury in High-Fat Diet and L-NAME-treated Rats," *European Journal of Nutrition* 51, no. 1 (2012): 57. DOI: 10.1007/s00394-011-0182-7.

38. P. Singh, "Chemical Profile, Antifungal, Antiaflatoxigenic and Antioxidant Activity of *Citrus maxima Burm.* and *Citrus sinensis (L.) Osbeck* Essential Oils and Their Cyclic Monoterpene, DL-limonene," *Food and Chemistry Toxicology* 48, no. 6 (2010): 1734–1740. DOI: 10.1016/j.fct.2010.04.001.

39. S. Asnaashari et al., "Essential Oil from *Citrus aurantifolia* Prevents Ketotifen-induced Weight-gain in Mice," *Phytotherapy Research* 24, no. 12 (2010): 1893–1897. DOI: 10.1002/ptr.3227.

40. P. A. d'Alessio et al., "Anti-stress Effects of d-Limonene and Its Metabolite Perillyl Alcohol," *Rejuvenation Research* 17, no. 2 (2014): 145–149. DOI: 10.1089/rej.2013.1515.

41. H. M. Park, "Limonene, a Natural Cyclic Terpene, Is an Agonistic Ligand for Adenosine A(2A) Receptors," *Biochemical and Biophysical Research Communications* 404, no. 1 (2011): 345–348. DOI: 10.1016/j.bbrc.2010.11.121.

42. R. Tisserand and R. Young, *Essential Oil Safety: A Guide for Health Care Professionals*, 2nd ed. (London: Churchill Livingstone, 2013), 580.

Chapter 8: HEAL YOURSELF

1. J. R. Santin et al., "Gastroprotective Activity of Essential Oil of the *Syzygium aromaticum* and Its Major Component Eugenol in Different Animal

Models," *Naunyn-Schmiedeberg's Archives of Phar-macology* 383, no. 2 (2011): 149–158. DOI: 10.1007/s00210-010-0582-x.

2. V. B. Liju, K. Jeena, and R. Kuttan, "Gastropro-tective Activity of Essential Oils from Turmeric and Ginger," *Journal of Basic and Clinical Physiology and Pharmacology* 26, no. 1 (2015): 95–103. DOI: 10.1515/jbcpp-2013-0165.

3. C. Canavan, J. West, and T. Card, "The Epidemi-ology of Irritable Bowel Syndrome," *Clinical Epi-demiology* 6 (2014): 71–80. DOI: 10.2147/CLEP.S40245.

4. A. C. Ford et al., "Effect of Fibre, Antispasmodics, and Peppermint Oil in the Treatment of Irritable Bowel Syndrome: Systematic Review and Meta-analysis," *BMJ* 337 (2008): a2313. DOI: 10.1136/bmj.a2313.

5. A. C. Dukowicz, B. E. Lacy, and G. M. Levine, "Small Intestinal Bacterial Overgrowth: A Compre-hensive Review," *Gastroenterology & Hepatology* 3, no. 2 (2007): 112–122.

6. S. Shipradeep et al., "Development of Probiotic Candidate in Combination with Essential Oils from Medicinal Plant and Their Effect on Enteric Pathogens: A Review," *Gastroenterology Research and Practice* 2012, ID no. 457150 (2012). DOI: 10.1155/2012/457150.

7. J. A. Hawrelak, T. Cattley, S. P. Myers, "Essential Oils in the Treatment of Intestinal Dysbiosis: A Preliminary in Vitro Study," *Alternative Medicine Review* 14, no. 4 (2009): 380–384.

8. S. C. Bischoff et al., "Intestinal Permeability—a New Target for Disease Prevention and Therapy," *BMC Gastroenterology* 14 (2014): 189. DOI: 10.1186/s12876-014-0189-7; M. C. Arrieta, L. Bistritz, and J. B. Meddings, "Alterations in Intestinal Perme-ability," *Gut* 55, no. 10 (2006): 1512–1520. DOI: 10.1136/gut.2005.085373.

9. Y. Zou et al., "Oregano Essential Oil Improves Intestinal Morphology and Expression of Tight Junction Proteins Associated with Modulation of Selected Intestinal Bacteria and Immune Status in a Pig Model," *BioMed Research International* 2016, ID no. 5436738 (2016). DOI: 10.1155/2016/5436738.

10. J. Dyer et al., "The Use of Aromasticks at a Can-cer Centre: A Retrospective Audit," *Complementary Therapies in Clinical Practice* 20, no. 4 (2013): 203–206; M. Navarra et al., "*Citrus bergamia* Essential Oil: From Basic Research to Clinical Application," *Frontiers in Pharmacology* 6, no. 36 (2015). DOI: 10.3389/fphar.2015.00036; J. H. Hwang, "The Effects of the Inhalation Method Using Essential Oils on Blood Pressure and Stress Responses of Cli-ents with Essential Hypertension," *Journal of Korean Academic Nursing* 36, no. 7 (2006): 1123–1134. DOI: 10.4040/jkan.2006.36.7.1123.

11. Dyer et al., "The Use of Aromasticks at a Cancer Centre: A Retrospective Audit."

12. F. Rashidi Fakari et al., "Effect of Inhalation of Aroma of Geranium Essence on Anxiety and Physi-ological Parameters During First Stage of Labor in Nulliparous Women: A Randomized Clinical Trial," *Journal of Caring Sciences* 4, no. 2 (2015): 135–141. DOI: 10.15171/jcs.2015.014.

13. J. K. Srivastava et al., "Chamomile: A Herbal Medi-cine of the Past with Bright Future," *Molecular Med-icine Reports* 3, no. 6 (2010): 895–901.

14. Hwang, "The Effects of the Inhalation Method Using Essential Oils on Blood Pressure and Stress Responses of Clients with Essential Hypertension"; Dyer et al., "The Use of Aromasticks at a Cancer Centre: A Retrospective Audit"; M. Keshavarz Afshar et al., "Lavender Fragrance Essential Oil and the Quality of Sleep in Postpartum Women," *Ira-nian Red Crescent Medical Journal* 17, no. 4 (2015): e25880. DOI: 10.5812/ircmj.17(4)2015.25880.

15. Dyer et al., "The Use of Aromasticks at a Cancer Centre: A Retrospective Audit."

16. S. Y. Choi et al., "Effects of Inhalation of Essential Oil of *Citrus aurantium* L. var. *amara* on Menopausal Symptoms, Stress, and Estrogen in Postmeno-pausal Women: A Randomized Controlled Trial," *Evidence-Based Complementary and Alternative Med-icine* 2014, ID no. 796518 (2014). DOI: 10.1155/2014/796518.

17. M. Igarashi et al., "Effects of Olfactory Stimula-tion with Rose and Orange Oil on Prefrontal Cor-tex Activity," *Complementary Therapies in Medicine*

22, no. 6 (2014): 1027–1031. DOI: 10.1016/j.ctim.2014.09.003.

18. B. F. M. T Andrade et al., "Effect of Inhaling *Cymbopogon martinii* Essential Oil and Geraniol on Serum Biochemistry Parameters and Oxidative Stress in Rats," *Biochemistry Research International* 2014, ID no. 493183 (2014). DOI: 10.1155/2014/493183.

19. Dyer et al., "The Use of Aromasticks at a Cancer Centre: A Retrospective Audit."

20. Igarashi et al., "Effects of Olfactory Stimulation with Rose and Orange Oil on Prefrontal Cortex Activity"; Y. Wu et al., "The Metabolic Responses to Aerial Diffusion of Essential Oils," *PLoS ONE* 7, no. 9 (2012): e44830. DOI: 10.1371/journal.pone.0044830.

21. H. Takemoto et al., "Sedative Effects of Vapor Inhalation of Agarwood Oil and Spikenard Extract and Identification of Their Active Components," *Journal of Natural Medicines* 62, no. 1 (2008): 41. DOI: 10.1007/s11418-007-0177-0.

22. D.-J. Jung et al., "Effects of Ylang-Ylang Aroma on Blood Pressure and Heart Rate in Healthy Men," *Journal of Exercise Rehabilitation* 9, no. 2 (2013): 250–255. DOI: 10.12965/jer.130007; Hwang, "The Effects of the Inhalation Method Using Essential Oils on Blood Pressure and Stress Responses of Clients with Essential Hypertension."

23. A. Bounihi et al., "*In Vivo* Potential Anti-Inflammatory Activity of *Melissa officinalis* L. Essential Oil," *Advances in Pharmacological Sciences* 2013, ID no. 101759 (2013). DOI: 10.1155/2013/101759.

24. S. Y. Chang, "Effects of Aroma Hand Massage on Pain, State Anxiety and Depression in Hospice Patients with Terminal Cancer," *Journal of Korean Academy of Nursing* 38, no. 4 (2008): 493–502. DOI: 10.4040/jkan.2008.38.4.493.

25. V. F. Veiga Junior et al., "Chemical Composition and Anti-inflammatory Activity of Copaiba Oils from *Copaifera cearensis* Huber ex Ducke, *Copaifera reticulata* Ducke and *Copaifera multijuga* Hayne—a Comparative Study," *Journal of Ethnopharmacology* 112, no. 2 (2007): 248–254; M.-C. Ou et al., "Pain Relief Assessment by Aromatic Essential Oil Massage on Outpatients with Primary Dysmenorrhea: A Randomized, Double-blind Clinical Trial,"

Journal of Obstetrics and Gynaecology Research 38, no. 5 (2012): 817–822. DOI: 10.1111/j.1447-0756.2011.01802.x.

26. S. Asnaashari et al., "Essential Oil from *Citrus aurantifolia* Prevents Ketotifen-induced Weight-Gain in Mice," *Phytotherapy Research* 24, no. 10 (2010): 1893–1897. DOI: 10.1002/ptr.3227.

27. H. J. Kim, "Effect of Aromatherapy Massage on Abdominal Fat and Body Image in Post-menopausal Women," *Taehan Kanho Hakhoe Chi* 37, no. 4 (2007): 603–612.

Chapter 9: PERSONAL CARE PRODUCTS

1. Environmental Working Group, "Body Burden: The Pollution in Newborns," July 14, 2005, http://www.ewg.org/research/body-burden-pollution-newborns, accessed April 17, 2017.

2. Ibid.

3. U.S. Food and Drug Administration, "FDA Issues Final Rule on Safety and Effectiveness of Antibacterial Soaps," September 16, 2016, https://www.fda.gov/NewsEvents/Newsroom/PressAnnouncements/ucm517478.htm, accessed April 14, 2017.

4. Ibid.

5. C. Ballantyne, "Strange But True: Antibacterial Products May Do More Harm Than Good," *Scientific American*, June 7, 2007; C. Rees et al., "The Impact of Bisphenol A and Triclosan on Immune Parameters in the U.S. Population, NHANES, 2003–2006," *Environmental Health Perspectives* 119, no. 3 (2011): 390–396. DOI: 10.1289/ehp.1002883.

6. G. Matiz et al., "Effectiveness of Antimicrobial Formulations for Acne Based on Orange (*Citrus sinensis*) and Sweet Basil (*Ocimum basilicum L.*) Essential Oils," *Biomedica* 32, no. 1 (2012): 125–133. DOI: 10.1590/S0120-41572012000100014.

7. Y. Zu et al., "Activities of Ten Essential Oils Towards *Propionibacterium acnes* and PC-3, A-549 and MCF-7 Cancer Cells," *Molecules* 15, no. 5 (2010): 3200–3210. DOI: 10.3390/molecules15053200.

8. G. Matiz et al., "Effectiveness of Antimicrobial Formulations for Acne Based on Orange (*Citrus sinensis*) and Sweet Basil (*Ocimum basilicum L.*) Essential Oils."

Chapter 10: AROUND THE HOUSE

1. National Research Council, Review of the Styrene Assessment in the National Toxicology Program 12th Report on Carcinogens (Washington, D.C.: National Academies Press, 2014), https://www.ncbi.nlm.nih.gov/books/NBK241556/.
2. B. E. Fisher, "Scents and Sensitivity," *Environmental Health Perspectives* 106, no. 12 (1998): 594–599.
3. International Fragrance Association, "Ingredients," http://www.ifraorg.org/en-us/ingredients#.WPER 24VGqTP, accessed April 14, 2017.

Chapter 11: ESSENTIAL OILS FOR ATHLETES

1. A. Fontinelle, "The Energy Drinks Industry," Investopedia, http://www.investopedia.com/articles/investing/022315/energy-drinks-industry.asp, accessed April 13, 2017.
2. S. M. Siefert et al., "Health Effects of Energy Drinks on Children, Adolescents, and Young Adults," *Pediatrics* 127, no. 3 (2011): 511–528. DOI: 10.1542/peds.2009-3592.
3. B. J. Wolk, M. Ganetsky, and K. M. Babu, "Toxicity of Energy Drinks," *Current Opinion in Pediatrics* 24, no. 2 (2012): 243–251. DOI: 10.1097/MOP.0b013 e3283506827; E. Matuszkiewicz, "Energy Drinks as a Cause of Seizures—Real or Possible Danger?" *Przeglad Lekarski* 72, no. 1 (2015): 42–44.
4. Ibid.
5. C. Rosenbloom, "Energy Drinks, Caffeine, and Athletes," *Nutrition Today* 49, no. 2 (2014): 49–54. DOI: http://10.1097/NT.0000000000000022.
6. Ibid.
7. C. J. Reissig, E. C. Strain, and R. R. Griffiths, "Caffeinated Energy Drinks—A Growing Problem," *Drug and Alcohol Dependence* 99, nos. 1–3 (2009): 1–10. DOI: 10.1016/j.drugalcdep.2008.08.001.
8. Ibid.; National Center for Complementary and Integrative Health, "Energy Drinks," https://nccih.nih.gov/health/energy-drinks, accessed April 13, 2017.
9. C. Alford, H. Cox, and R. Wescott, "The Effects of Red Bull Energy Drink on Human Performance and Mood," *Amino Acids* 21, no. 2 (2001): 139–150.
10. D. G. Candow, "Effect of Sugar-free Red Bull Energy Drink on High-intensity Run Time-to-Exhaustion in Young Adults," *Journal of Strength and Conditioning Research* 23, no. 4 (2009): 1271–1275. DOI: 10.1519/JSC.0b013e3181a026c2.
11. J. M. Eckerson, "Acute Ingestion of Sugar-free Red Bull Energy Drink Has No Effect on Upper Body Strength and Muscular Endurance in Resistance Trained Men," *Journal of Strength and Conditioning Research* 27, no. 8 (2013): 2248–2254. DOI: 10.1519/JSC.0b013e31827e14f2.
12. Reissig, Strain, and Griffiths, "Caffeinated Energy Drinks—A Growing Problem."
13. National Center for Complementary and Integrative Health, "Energy Drinks"; O. P. Wójcik et al., "The Potential Protective Effects of Taurine on Coronary Heart Disease," *Atherosclerosis* 208, no. 1 (2010): 19. DOI: 10.1016/j.atherosclerosis.2009.06.002.
14. Ibid.; Y.-J. Xu, "The Potential Health Benefits of Taurine in Cardiovascular Disease," *Experimental & Clinical Cardiology* 13, no. 2 (2008): 57–65; A. Shao and J. N. Hathcock, "Risk Assessment for the Amino Acids Taurine, L-glutamine and L-arginine," *Regulatory Toxicology and Pharmacology* 50, no. 3 (2008): 376–399. DOI: 10.1016/j.yrtph.2008.01.004.
15. K. Zeratsky, "Taurine Is Listed as an Ingredient in Many Energy Drinks. What Is Taurine? Is it Safe?" Nutrition and Healthy Eating, Mayo Clinic, http://www.mayoclinic.org/healthy-lifestyle/nutrition-and-healthy-eating/expert-answers/taurine/faq-20058177, accessed April 13, 2017.
16. J. P. Higgins, T. D. Tuttle, and C. L. Higgins, "Energy Beverages: Content and Safety," *Mayo Clinic Proceedings* 85, no. 11 (2010): 1033–1041. DOI: 10.4065/mcp.2010.038.
17. M. R. Beyranvand et al., "Effect of Taurine Supplementation on Exercise Capacity of Patients with Heart Failure," *Journal of Cardiology* 57, no. 3 (2011): 333–337. DOI: 10.1016/j.jjcc.2011.01.007.
18. B. J. Wolk, M. Ganetsky, and K. M. Babu, "Toxicity of Energy Drinks," *Current Opinion in Pediatrics*, 24, no. 2 (2012): 243–251. DOI: 10.1097/MOP.0b013e3283506827.
19. A. Meamarbashi and A. Rajabi, "The Effects of Peppermint on Exercise Performance," *Journal of the International Society of Sports Nutrition* 10 (2013): 15.

DOI: 10.1186/1550-2783-10-15; A. Meamarbashi, "Instant Effects of Peppermint Essential Oil on the Physiological Parameters and Exercise Performance," *Avicenna Journal of Phytomedicine* 4, no. 1 (2014): 72–78.

20. Meamarbashi and Rajabi, "The Effects of Peppermint on Exercise Performance"; Meamarbashi, "Instant Effects of Peppermint Essential Oil on the Physiological Parameters and Exercise Performance."

21. Meamarbashi and Rajabi, "The Effects of Peppermint on Exercise Performance."

22. S. K. Yeap et al., "Antistress and Antioxidant Effects of Virgin Coconut Oil *in vivo*," *Experimental and Therapeutic Medicine* 9, no. 1 (2015): 39–42. DOI: 10.3892/etm.2014.2045.

23. M.-C. Ou et al., "The Effectiveness of Essential Oils for Patients with Neck Pain: A Randomized Controlled Study," *Journal of Alternative Complementary Medicine* 20, no. 10 (2014): 771–779. DOI: 10.1089/acm.2013.0453.

24. A. Babar, "Essential Oils Used in Aromatherapy: A Systemic Review," *Asian Pacific Journal of Tropical Biomedicine* 5, no. 8 (2015): 601–611. DOI: 10.1016/j.apjtb.2015.05.007.

25. Ayurvedic Oils, "Fir Needle Oil," http://ayurvedicoils.com/tag/fir-needle-essential-oil, accessed April 13, 2017.

Part 3: WOMEN'S HEALTH

1. Y. Wang, et al., "Do Men Consult Less Than Women? An Analysis of Routinely Collected UK General Practice Data," *BMJ Open*, 3, no. 8 (2013): e003320. DOI: 10.1136/bmjopen-2013-003320.

2. E. J. Bartley and R. B. Fillingim, "Sex Differences in Pain: A Brief Review of Clinical and Experimental Findings," *BJA: British Journal of Anaesthesia* 111, no. 1 (2013): 52–58. DOI: 10.1093/bja/aet127.

3. M. Altemus, N. Sarvaiya, and C. N. Epperson, "Sex Differences in Anxiety and Depression Clinical Perspectives," *Frontiers in Neuroendocrinology* 35, no. 3 (2014): 320–330. DOI: 10.1016/j.yfrne.2014.05.004.

4. E. C. Suarez, "Self-Reported Symptoms of Sleep Disturbance and Inflammation, Coagulation, Insulin Resistance and Psychosocial Distress: Evidence for Gender Disparity," *Brain, Behavior, and Immunity* 22, no. 6 (2008): 960–968. DOI: 10.1016/j.bbi.2008.01.011; K. C. Smith, "Sex, Gender, and Health," Johns Hopkins Bloomberg School of Public Health, 2006, http://ocw.jhsph.edu/courses/SocialBehavioralAspectsPublicHealth/PDFs/Unit2Gender.pdf, accessed March 21, 2017.

5. V. Regitz-Zagrosek, "Sex and Gender Differences in Health: Science and Society Series on Sex and Science," *EMBO Reports* 13, no. 7 (2012): 596–603. DOI: 10.1038/embor.2012.87.

6. R. C. Rabin, "The Drug-Dose Gender Gap," *Well* (blog), NYTimes.com, January 28, 2013, https://well.blogs.nytimes.com/2013/01/28/the-drug-dose-gender-gap, accessed March 21, 2017.

Chapter 13: PREMENSTRUAL SYNDROME

1. P. S. O'Brien, P. M. Shaughn, and K. M. K. Ismail, "History of the Premenstrual Disorders," in *The Premenstrual Syndromes: PMS and PMDD*, eds. P. M. S. O'Brien, A. J. Rapkin, and P. J. Schmidt (London: Informa Healthcare, 2007), 1–8.

2. R. Greene and K. Dalton, "The Premenstrual Syndrome, *British Medical Journal* 1, no. 4818 (1953): 1007–1014.

3. C. N. Epperson and L. V. Hantsoo, "Making Strides to Simplify Diagnosis of Premenstrual Dysphoric Disorder," *American Journal of Psychiatry* 174, no. 1 (2017): 6–7. DOI: 10.1176/appi.ajp.2016.16101144.

4. P. Sasannejad et al., "Lavender Essential Oil in the Treatment of Migraine Headache: A Placebo-Controlled Clinical Trial," *European Neurology* 67, no. 5 (2012): 288–291. DOI: 10.1159/000335249.

5. M.-H. Hur, M. S. Lee, K.-Y. Seong, and M.-K. Lee, "Aromatherapy Massage on the Abdomen for Alleviating Menstrual Pain in High School Girls: A Preliminary Controlled Clinical Study," *Evidence-Based Complementary and Alternative Medicine* 2012, ID no. 187163 (2012). DOI: 10.1155/2012/187163.

6. M.-C. Ou, T-F. Hsu, A. C. Lai, and Y.-T. Lin, "Pain Relief Assessment by Aromatic Essential Oil Massage on Outpatients with Primary Dysmenorrhea: A Randomized, Double-blind Clinical Trial,"

Journal of Obstetrics and Gynaecology 38, no. 5 (2012): 817. DOI: 10.1111/j.1447-0756.2011.01802.x.

7. S. N. Ostad et al., "The Effect of Fennel Essential Oil on Uterine Contraction as a Model for Dysmenorrhea, Pharmacology and Toxicology Study," *Journal of Ethnopharmacology* 76, no. 3 (2001): 299–304.

8. J. Silva et al., "Analgesic and Anti-inflammatory Effects of Essential Oils of Eucalyptus," *Journal of Ethnopharmacology* 89, nos. 2–3 (2003): 277–283. DOI: 10.1016/j.jep.2003.09.007.

9. J. A. Reed, J. Almeida, B. Wershing, and B. Raudenbush, "Effects of Peppermint Scent on Appetite Control and Caloric Intake," *Appetite* 51, no. 2 (2008): 393. DOI: 10.1016/j.appet.2008.04.196.

10. M. Igarashi et al., "Effects of Olfactory Stimulation with Rose and Orange Oil on Prefrontal Cortex Activity," *Complementary Therapies in Medicine* 22, no. 6 (2014): 1027–1031. DOI: 10.1016/j.ctim.2014.09.003.

11. S. Y. Choi et al., "Effects of Inhalation of Essential Oil of *Citrus aurantium* L. var. *amara* on Menopausal Symptoms, Stress, and Estrogen in Postmenopausal Women: A Randomized Controlled Trial," *Evidence-Based Complementary and Alternative Medicine* 2014, ID no. 796518 (2014). DOI: 10.1155/2014/796518.

12. S. Holt, "Natural Approaches to Promote Sexual Function, Part 2: Stimulants and Dietary Supplements," *Alternative and Complementary Therapies* 5, no. 5 (1999): 279–285.

13. M.-H. Hur, Y. S. Yang, and M. S. Lee, "Aromatherapy Massage Affects Menopausal Symptoms in Korean Climacteric Women: A Pilot-Controlled Clinical Trial," *Evidence-Based Complementary and Alternative Medicine* 5, no. 3 (2008): 325–328. DOI: 10.1093/ecam/nem027.

14. T. Hongratanaworakit, "Relaxing Effect of Rose Oil on Humans," *Natural Product Communications* 4, no. 2 (2009): 291–296.

15. M.-C. Ou et al., "Pain Relief Assessment by Aromatic Essential Oil Massage on Outpatients with Primary Dysmenorrhea."

16. S. H. Han et al., "Effect of Aromatherapy on Symptoms of Dysmenorrhea in College Students: A Randomized Placebo-controlled Clinical Trial," *Journal of Alternative and Complementary Medicine* 12, no. 6 (2006): 535–541.

Chapter 14: FERTILITY, PREGNANCY, LABOR, POSTPARTUM, AND NURSING

1. Eunice Kennedy Shriver National Institute of Child Health and Human Development, "How Common Is Male Infertility and What Are Its Causes?" National Institutes of Health, https://www.nichd.nih.gov/health/topics/menshealth/conditioninfo/Pages/infertility.aspx#f4, accessed March 23, 2017.

2. A. Agarwal, S. Prabakaran, and S. S. Allamaneni, "Relationship Between Oxidative Stress, Varicocele and Infertility: A Meta-analysis," *Reproductive Biomedicine Online* 12, no. 5 (2006): 630–633.

3. T. Safarnavadeh and M. Rastegarpanah, "Antioxidants and Infertility Treatment, the Role of *Satureja Khuzestanica*: A Mini Systematic Review," *Iranian Journal of Reproductive Medicine* 9, no. 2 (2011): 61–70.

4. E. Burns, "An Investigation into the Use of Aromatherapy in Intrapartum Midwifery Practice," *Journal of Alternative and Complementary Medicine* 6, no. 2 (2000): 141–147.

5. E. Burns et al., "Aromatherapy in Childbirth: A Pilot Randomised Controlled Trial," *BJOG: An International Journal of Obstetrics and Gynaecology* 114, no. 7 (2007): 838–844.

6. E. Burns et al., "The Use of Aromatherapy in Intrapartum Midwifery Practice an Observational Study," *Complementary Therapies in Nursing and Midwifery* 6, no. 1 (2000): 33–34.

7. M. Namazi et al., "Effects of *Citrus aurantium* (Bitter Orange) on the Severity of First-Stage Labor Pain," *Iranian Journal of Pharmaceutical Research* 13, no. 3 (2014): 1011–1018.

8. F. Rashidi Fakari, M. Tabatabaeichehr, and H. Mortazavi, "The Effect of Aromatherapy by Essential Oil of Orange on Anxiety During Labor: A Randomized Clinical Trial," *Iranian Journal of Nursing and Midwifery Research* 20, no. 6 (2015): 661–664. DOI: 10.4103/1735-9066.170001.

9. F. Rashidi Fakari et al., "Effect of Inhalation of

Aroma of Geranium Essence on Anxiety and Physiological Parameters During First Stage of Labor in Nulliparous Women: A Randomized Clinical Trial," *Journal of Caring Sciences* 4, no. 2 (2015): 135–141. DOI: 10.15171/jcs.2015.014.

10. M. Kheirkhah et al., "Comparing the Effects of Aromatherapy with Rose Oils and Warm Foot Bath on Anxiety in the First Stage of Labor in Nulliparous Women," *Iranian Red Crescent Medical Journal* 16, no. 9 (2014): e14455. DOI: 10.5812/ircmj.

11. P. H. Koulivand, M. Khaleghi Ghadiri, and A. Gorji, "Lavender and the Nervous System," *Evidence-Based Complementary and Alternative Medicine* 2013, ID no. 681304 (2013). DOI: 10.1155/2013/681304.

12. M. Kaviani et al., "Comparison of the Effect of Aromatherapy with *Jasminum officinale* and *Salvia officinale* on Pain Severity and Labor Outcome in Nulliparous Women," *Iranian Journal of Nursing and Midwifery Research* 19, no. 6 (2014): 666–672.

13. M. Erick, "Morning Sickness Impact Study," *Midwifery Today with International Midwife*, no. 59 (2001): 30–32.

14. P. Yavari kia et al., "The Effect of Lemon Inhalation Aromatherapy on Nausea and Vomiting of Pregnancy: A Double-Blinded, Randomized, Controlled Clinical Trial," *Iranian Red Crescent Medical Journal* 16, no. 3 (2014): e14360. DOI:10.5812/ircmj.14360.

15. M. H. Hur and M. H. Park, "Effects of Aromatherapy on Labor Process, Labor Pain, Labor Stress Response and Neonatal Status of Primipara: Randomized Clinical Trial," *Korean Journal of Obstetrics & Gynecol*ogy 46, no. 4 (2003): 776–783.

16. L. Gori et al., "Can Estragole in Fennel Seed Decoctions Really Be Considered a Danger for Human Health? A Fennel Safety Update," *Evidence-Based Complementary and Alternative Medicine* 2012, ID no. 860542 (2012). DOI: 10.1155/2012/860542.

17. L. Rosti et al., "Toxic Effects of a Herbal Tea Mixture in Two Newborns," *Acta Paediatrica* 83, no. 6 (1994): 683.

18. S. Fayazi, M. Babashahi, and M. Rezaei, "The Effect of Inhalation Aromatherapy on Anxiety Level of the Patients in Preoperative Period," *Iranian Journal of Nursing and Midwifery Research* 16, no. 4 (2011): 278–283; Kaviani et al., "Comparison of the Effect of Aromatherapy with *Jasminum officinale* and *Salvia officinale* on Pain Severity and Labor Outcome in Nulliparous Women."

19. National Association of Holistic Aromatherapy, "Exploring Aromatherapy: Safety Information, Pregnancy Safety," http://naha.org/index.php/explore-aromatherapy/safety/#pregnancy, accessed March 25, 2017.

20. M. H. Hur and S. H. Han, "Clinical Trial of Aromatherapy on Postpartum Mother's Perineal Healing," *Taehan Kanho Hakhoe Chi* 34, no. 1 (2004): 53–62.

21. K. L. Wisner et al., "Onset Timing, Thoughts of Self-harm, and Diagnoses in Postpartum Women with Screen-Positive Depression Findings," *JAMA Psychiatry* 70, no. 5 (2013): 490–498. DOI: 10.1001/jamapsychiatry.2013.87.

Chapter 15: CANDIDA

1. M. Solomon, A. M. Itsekson, and A. Lev-Sagie, "Autoimmune Progesterone Dermatitis," *Current Dermatology Reports* 2, no. 4 (2013): 258–263.

2. Centers for Disease Control and Prevention, "Candidiasis," https://www.cdc.gov/fungal/diseases/candidiasis/, accessed March 25, 2017.

3. Ibid.

4. National Health Service, "Vaginal Thrush," http://www.nhs.uk/conditions/thrush/Pages/Introduction.aspx, accessed March 25, 2017; D. Sanglard, "Emerging Threats in Antifungal-Resistant Fungal Pathogens," *Frontiers in Medicine* 3, no. 11 (2016). DOI: 10.3389/fmed.2016.00011.

5. R. S. Pereira et al., "Antibacterial Activity of Essential Oils on Microorganisms Isolated from Urinary Tract Infections," *Revista de Saude Publica* 38, no. 2 (2004): 326–328.

6. M. H. Lodhia et al., "Antibacterial Activity of Essential Oils from Palmarosa, Evening Primrose, Lavender and Tuberose," *Indian Journal of Pharmaceutical Sciences* 71, no. 2 (2009): 134–136. DOI: 10.4103/0250-474X.54278.

7. R. Sender, S. Fuchs, and R. Milo, "Revised Estimates for the Number of Human and Bacteria

Cells in the Body," *PLoS Biology* 14, no. 8 (2016): e1002533, DOI:10.1371/journal.pbio.1002533.

8. V. Oliveira Carvalho, "The New Mutation L321F in *Candida albicans* ERG11 Gene May Be Associated with Fluconazole Resistance," *Revista Iberoamericana Micologia* 30, no. 3 (2013): 209–212. DOI: 10.1016/j.riam.2013.01.001.

9. U.S. Food & Drug Administration, "FDA Advises Restricting Fluoroquinolone Antibiotic Use for Certain Uncomplicated Infections; Warns About Disabling Side Effects That Can Occur Together," https://www.fda.gov/Drugs/DrugSafety/ucm500 143.htm, accessed March 25, 2017.

10. P. Nenoff, U. F. Haustein, and W. Brandt, "Antifungal Activity of the Essential Oil of *Melaleuca alternifolia* (Tea Tree Oil) Against Pathogenic Fungi in Vitro," *Skin Pharmacology* 9, no. 6 (1996): 388–394.

11. J. Buckle, *Clinical Aromatherapy,* 3rd ed. (London: Churchill Livingstone, 2014), 386.

12. J. Irish et al., "Honey Has an Antifungal Effect Against *Candida* Species," *Medical Mycology* 44, no. 3 (2006): 289–291. DOI: 10.1080/13693780500417037.

13. M. Darvishi et al., "The Comparison of Vaginal Cream of Mixing Yogurt, Honey and Clotrimazole on Symptoms of Vaginal Candidiasis," *Global Journal of Health Science* 7, no. 6 (2015): 108–116. DOI: 10.5539/gjhs.v7n6p108.

14. F. Behmanesh et al., "Antifungal Effect of Lavender Essential Oil (*Lavandula angustifolia*) and Clotrimazole on *Candida albicans*: An *In Vitro* Study," *Scientifica* (2015): 261397. DOI: 10.1155/2015/261397.

15. K. Rajkowska et al., "The Effect of Thyme and Tea Tree Oils on Morphology and Metabolism of Candida albicans," *Acta Biochimica Polonica* 61, no. 2 (2014): 305–310.

16. V. Agarwal, P. Lal, and V. Pruthi, "Effect of Plant Oils on *Candida albicans*," *Journal of Microbiology, Immunology and Infection* 43, no. 5 (2010): 447–451. DOI: 10.1016/S1684-1182(10)60069-2.

17. N. Maruyama et al., "Protective Activity of Geranium Oil and Its Component, Geraniol, in Combination with Vaginal Washing Against Vaginal Candidiasis in Mice," *Biological and Pharmaceutical Bulletin* 31, no. 8 (2008): 1501–1506.

18. P. H. Warnke et al., "The Battle Against Multiresistant Strains: Renaissance of Antimicrobial Essential Oils as a Promising Force to Fight Hospital-Acquired Infections," *Journal of Cranio-Maxillo-Facial Surgery* 37, no. 7 (2009): 392–397. DOI: 10.1016/j.jcms.2009.03.017.

19. M. Białoń et al., "The Influence of Chemical Composition of Commercial Lemon Essential Oils on the Growth of *Candida* Strains," *Mycopathologia* 177, nos. 1–2 (2014): 29–39. DOI: 10.1007/s11046-013 -9723-3.

20. E. Pinto et al., "Antifungal Activity of the Clove Essential Oil from *Syzygium aromaticum* on *Candida, Aspergillus* and Dermatophyte Species," *Journal of Medical Microbiology* 58 (2009): 1454–1462. DOI: 10.1099/jmm.0.010538-0.

21. S. Tadtong et al., "Antimicrobial Activity of Blended Essential Oil Preparation," *Natural Product Communication* 7, no. 10 (2012): 1401–1404.

22. Buckle, *Clinical Aromatherapy,* 386.

23. Ibid.

Chapter 16: AUTOIMMUNITY

1. C. A. Siegel et al., "Risk of Lymphoma Associated with Combination Anti-Tumor Necrosis Factor and Immunomodulator Therapy for the Treatment of Crohn's Disease: A Meta-Analysis," *Clinical Gastroenterology and Hepatology* 7, no. 8 (2009): 874–881. DOI: 10.1016/j.cgh.2009.01.004.

2. American Autoimmune Related Diseases Association, "Autoimmune Disease Statistics," https://www.aarda.org/news-information/statistics, accessed March 26, 2017.

3. National Institute of Allergies and Infectious Diseases, "Gender-Specific Health Challenges Facing Women," https://www.niaid.nih.gov/research/gender -specific-health-challenges, accessed March 27, 2017.

4. J. E. Gudjonsson et al., "A Gene Network Regulated by the Transcription Factor VGLL3 as a Promoter of Sex-Biased Autoimmune Diseases," *Nature Immunology* 18 (2017): 152–160. DOI: 10.1038/ni.3643.

5. D. Nakazawa, *The Autoimmune Epidemic* (New York: Simon & Schuster, 2008).

6. Ibid.

7. J. Buckle, *Clinical Aromatherapy,* 3rd ed. (London: Churchill Livingstone, 2014).

8. B. Adam et al., "A Combination of Peppermint Oil and Caraway Oil Attenuates the Post-Inflammatory Visceral Hyperalgesia in a Rat Model," *Scandinavian Journal of Gastroenterology* 41, no. 2 (2006): 155–160. DOI: 10.1080/00365520500206442.

9. Y. A. Taher et al., "Experimental Evaluation of Anti-inflammatory, Antinociceptive and Antipyretic Activities of Clove Oil in Mice," *Libyan Journal of Medicine* 10 (2015). DOI: 10.3402/ljm.v10.28685.

10. J. Silva et al., "Analgesic and Anti-inflammatory Effects of Essential Oils of Eucalyptus," *Journal of Ethnopharmacology* 89, nos. 2–3 (2003): 277–283. DOI: 10.1016/j.jep.2003.09.007.

11. K. Jeena, V. B. Liju, and R. Kuttan, "Antioxidant, Anti-inflammatory and Antinociceptive Activities of Essential Oil from Ginger," *Indian Journal of Physiology and Pharmacology* 57, no. 1 (2013): 51–62.

12. G. L. Da Silva et al., "Antioxidant, Analgesic and Anti-inflammatory Effects of Lavender Essential Oil," *Anais da Academia Brasileira de Ciências* 87, no. 2 (2015): 1397–1408. DOI: 10.1590/0001 -3765201520150056.

13. O. Ming-Chiu et al., "The Effectiveness of Essential Oils for Patients with Neck Pain: A Randomized Controlled Study," *Journal of Alternative and Complementary Medicine* 20, no. 10 (2014): 771–779. DOI: 10.1089/acm.2013.0453.

14. A. Bukovská et al., "Effects of a Combination of Thyme and Oregano Essential Oils on TNBS-Induced Colitis in Mice," *Mediators of Inflammation* 2007, ID no. 23296 (2007). DOI: 10.1155 /2007/23296.

15. Z. Sun et al., "Chemical Composition and Anti-Inflammatory, Cytotoxic and Antioxidant Activities of Essential Oil from Leaves of *Mentha piperita* Grown in China," *PLoS ONE* 9, no. 12 (2014): e114767. DOI: 10.1371/journal.pone.0114767.

16. University of Maryland Medical Center, "Roman Chamomile," https://umm.edu/health/medical/alt med/herb/roman-chamomile, accessed March 27, 2017.

17. K. J. Koh et al., "Tea Tree Oil Reduces Histamine-induced Skin Inflammation," *British Journal of Dermatology* 147 (2002): 1212–1217. DOI: 10.1046 /j.1365-2133.2002.05034.x.

18. Bukovská et al., "Effects of a Combination of Thyme and Oregano Essential Oils on TNBS-Induced Colitis in Mice."

19. V. B. Liju, K. Jeena, and R. Kuttan, "An Evaluation of Antioxidant, Anti-inflammatory, and Antinociceptive Activities of Essential Oil from *Curcuma longa.* L," *Indian Journal of Pharmacology* 43, no. 5 (2011): 526–531. DOI: 10.4103/0253-7613.8496.

20. B. Adam et al., "A Combination of Peppermint Oil and Caraway Oil Attenuates the Post-inflammatory Visceral Hyperalgesia in a Rat Model."

21. Bukovská et al., "Effects of a Combination of Thyme and Oregano Essential Oils on TNBS-Induced Colitis in Mice."

22. F. A. Santos et al., "1,8-cineole (Eucalyptol), a Monoterpene Oxide Attenuates the Colonic Damage in Rats on Acute TNBS-colitis," *Food and Chemical Toxicology* 42, no. 4 (2004): 579–584. DOI: 10.1016/j.fct.2003.11.001.

23. R. Tisserand and R. Young, *Essential Oil Safety: A Guide for Health Care Professionals,* 2nd ed. (London: Churchill Livingstone, 2013).

24. F. Namjooyan et al., "Uses of Complementary and Alternative Medicine in Multiple Sclerosis," *Journal of Traditional and Complementary Medicine* 4, no. 3 (2014): 145–152. DOI: 10.4103/2225-4110.136543.

25. M. J. Kim, E. S. Nam, and S. I. Paik, "The Effects of Aromatherapy on Pain, Depression, and Life Satisfaction of Arthritis Patients," *Taehan Kanho Hakhoe Chi* 35, no. 1 (2005): 186–194.

26. J. L. Funk et al., "Anti-Arthritic Effects and Toxicity of the Essential Oils of Turmeric (*Curcuma longa* L.)," *Journal of Agricultural and Food Chemistry* 58, no. 2 (2010): 842–849. DOI: 10.1021/jf9027206.

Chapter 17: PERIMENOPAUSE, MENOPAUSE, AND POSTMENOPAUSE

1. Healthline, "Menopause by the Numbers: Facts, Statistics, and You," http://www.healthline.com/health /menopause/facts-statistics-infographic#2, accessed March 29, 2017; Mayo Clinic, "Perimenopause:

Symptoms and Causes," http://www.mayoclinic.org/diseases-conditions/perimenopause/symptoms-causes/dxc-20253775, accessed March 29, 2017.

2. B. Chopin Lucks, "Vitex agnus castus Essential Oil and Menopausal Balance: A Research Update," *Complementary Therapies in Nursing and Midwifery* 9, no. 3 (2003): 157–160.

3. M.-H. Hur, Y. S. Yang, and M. S. Lee, "Aromatherapy Massage Affects Menopausal Symptoms in Korean Climacteric Women: A Pilot-Controlled Clinical Trial," *Evidence-Based Complementary and Alternative Medicine* 5, no. 3 (2008): 325–328. DOI: 10.1093/ecam/nem027.

4. K.-B. Lee, E. Cho, and Y. S. Kang, "Changes in 5-hydroxytryptamine and Cortisol Plasma Levels in Menopausal Women After Inhalation of Clary Sage Oil," *Phytotherapy Research* 28 (2014): 1599–1605. DOI: 10.1002/ptr.5163.

5. University of Maryland Medical Center, "Lavender," http://umm.edu/health/medical/altmed/herb/lavender, accessed March 29, 2017.

6. L. Rafsanjani et al., "Comparison of the Efficacy of Massage and Aromatherapy Massage with Geranium on Depression in Postmenopausal Women: A Clinical Trial," *Zahedan Journal of Research in Medical Sciences* 17, no. 4 (2015): 1. DOI: 10.5812/zjrms.17(4)2015.970.

7. B. C. Lucks, J. Sørensen, and L. Veal, "Vitex agnus-castus Essential Oil and Menopausal Balance: A Self-care Survey," *Complementary Therapies in Nursing and Midwifery* 8, no. 3 (2002): 148–154. DOI: 10.1054/ctnm.2002.0634.

8. P. K. Dalal and M. Agarwal, "Postmenopausal Syndrome," *Indian Journal of Psychiatry* 57, Suppl. 2 (2015): S222–S232. DOI: 10.4103/0019-5545.161483.

9. Ibid.

10. S. Y. Choi, P. Kang, H. S. Lee, and G. H. Seol, "Effects of Inhalation of Essential Oil of *Citrus aurantium* L. var. *amara* on Menopausal Symptoms, Stress, and Estrogen in Postmenopausal Women: A Randomized Controlled Trial," *Evidence-Based Complementary and Alternative Medicine* 2014, ID no. 796518 (2014). DOI: 10.1155/2014/796518.

11. B. Ali, "Essential Oils Used in Aromatherapy: A Systemic Review," *Asian Pacific Journal of Tropical Biomedicine* 5, no. 8 (2015): 601–611. DOI: 10.1016/j.apjtb.2015.05.007.

12. H. J. Kim, "Effect of Aromatherapy Massage on Abdominal Fat and Body Image in Post-menopausal Women," *Taehan Kanho Hakhoe Chi* 37, no. 4 (2007): 603–612.

13. Mayo Clinic, "Menopause," http://www.mayoclinic.org/diseases-conditions/menopause/basics/definition/con-20019726, accessed March 29, 2017.

14. R. C Mühlbauer, "Common Herbs, Essential Oils, and Monoterpenes Potently Modulate Bone Metabolism," *Bone* 32, no. 4 (2003): 372–380. DOI: 10.1016/S8756-3282(03)00027-9.

RECOMMENDED RESOURCES

I have created several resources to help you on your journey to mastering the safe and therapeutic use of essential oils. If you have any questions or a testimonial you'd like to share, please contact me at: EssentialOils@DrEricZ.com

I always love to read the healing stories that flow through my inbox, telling me how essential oils have changed people's lives!

Healing Power of Essential Oils Demo Videos
- HealingPowerOfEssentialOils.com

http://DrEricZ.com (one of the most visited nonbranded essential oil databases online)

Dr. Z's Essential Oils Club
- Free Essential Oils Starter Kit
- http://drericz.com/eo-starterkit

Dr. Z's Inner Circle
- Essential Oils Education Membership (monthly subscription) http://EssentialOilsClub.info

Dr. Z's Essential Oil eCourses
- http://DrEricZ.com/Programs

Aromatherapy and Essential Products
- http://Store.DrEricZ.com—diffusers, wraps, bottles, carrying cases, pillow pets for kids, and more!
- http://www.amazon.com—an excellent resource for empty containers to hold your oil blends, including lotion dispensers, spritz bottles, and even stick deodorant containers.

Aromatherapy Reference Books, Texts, and Certification Courses
- *375 Essential Oils and Hydrosols.* Jeanne Rose.
- *Aromatherapy for Health Professionals,* 4th edition. Shirley Price and Len Price.
- Aromatherapy Practitioner Course. Atlantic Institute of Aromatherapy.
- *Aromatherapy Practitioner Reference Manual.* Sylla Sheppard-Hanger.
- *Clinical Aromatherapy: Essential Oils in Healthcare,* 3rd edition. Jane Buckle.
- *Essential Oil Chem 101.* Essential Oils University. Robert Pappas.
- *Essential Oil Safety: A Guide for Health Care Professionals,* 2nd edition. Robert Tisserand and Rodney Young.
- *Understanding Hydrolats: The Specific Hydrosols for Aromatherapy: A Guide for Health Professionals.* Len Price and Shirley Price.

Health and Safety Guides, Environmental Working Group
- EWG's Skin Deep Cosmetics Database— http://www.ewg.org/skindeep
- EWG's Guide to Healthy Cleaning— http://www.ewg.org/guides/cleaners
- EWG's Food Scores— http://www.ewg.org/foodscores

INDEX

absolutes, 18, 19, 20, 21

acne, 74, 155–56

ADHD, 67, 81, 104

adverse reactions. *See* safety considerations; *specific oils*

affirmations, 246

alcohol, as solvent, 22, 46

allergic reactions (to oils), 29, 40

allergies, 67, 180, 230

almond oil, 42, 43

aloe vera oil, 46

Alzheimer's disease, 108

amyris, 89

anethole, 31, 218–19, 250

angelica, 54, 89, 263

animals, 177–87
  basics and safety, 177–80, 182–83
  common problems, 180–81
  how to administer oils, 183–84, 187
  recipes, 181–82, 185–87

anise, 50, 193, 218–19, 250

anointing blend, 50

anti-aging body butter, 151–52

antibacterial cleansers. *See* cleansers; hand and body cleansers

antibacterial oils. *See* antimicrobial oils

antibiotic medications, 232–33

antidepressant oils. *See* depression; mood enhancement

antifungal medications, 232–33, 237

antifungal oils, 74, 75, 102, 103, 104, 164, 233. *See also* antimicrobial oils; candida

anti-inflammatory oils, 70, 72, 75, 102–3, 104, 111. *See also* pain relief
  for autoimmune conditions, 250–52, 255, 258
  inflammation-soothing roll-on or capsules, 251–52
  for pain relief, 84–85, 104, 110

antimicrobial oils, 64, 68, 69, 102–3. *See also* candida; cleansers; infections
  for acne, 155–56
  antibiotic ointment, 174–75
  citrus oils as, 59–60, 70, 102, 110–11, 155–56, 164
  foodborne illness and, 57
  oil pulling with, 59–60
  tea tree oil as, 74, 75
  for urinary tract infections, 232

antioxidant oils, 63, 70, 75, 102–3, 111, 206

antiviral oils, 68, 103

anxiety
  in animals, 180, 181–82
  anxiety inhaler, 109
  oils for, 72, 75–76, 80, 103, 104, 128, 200, 201
  PMS- or sex-related, 200, 201, 202
  pregnancy and birth-related, 208–9, 211, 212, 225

APD (autoimmune progesterone dermatitis), 228

aphrodisiacs. *See* libido

appetite, 83, 111, 199. *See also* cravings; weight loss

apricot oil, 42

Aromatherapie: The Essential Oils—Vegetable Hormones (Gattefossé), 16

aromatherapy basics. *See* essential oils basics; tools and techniques

artificial fragrances, 158

athletes, 167–76
  antibiotic ointment, 174–75
  energy drink dangers, 167–70
  muscle ache relief, 173–74
  performance boosters for, 171–73

autoimmune conditions, 84, 228, 245–58
  anti-inflammatory oils and blends, 250–52
  autoimmune progesterone dermatitis, 228
  basics, 245–47
  chronic inflammation and, 247–48
  essential oils research, 248–49, 252
  hypothyroidism, 189–91
  immunosuppressant medications, 245, 246, 247, 250
  multiple sclerosis, 255–56
  recipes, 251–52, 254–55, 256, 257–58
  rheumatoid arthritis, 257–58
  safety considerations, 249–50
  ulcerative colitis, 253–55

Avicenna, 16

avocado oil, 42

bacterial infections. *See* antimicrobial oils; infections

balsam/white fir, 85, 180. *See also* fir needle oils

About the Author

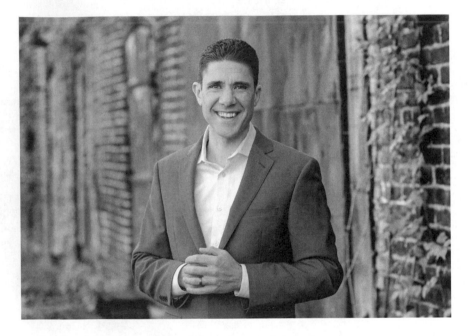

ERIC ZIELINSKI, D.C., has pioneered natural living and biblical health education since 2003. Trained as an aromatherapist, public health researcher, and chiropractor, Dr. Z started DrEricZ.com in 2014 to help people learn how to use natural remedies like essential oils safely and effectively. Now visited by more than four million natural health seekers every year, it has rapidly become the number one source for biblical health and non-branded essential oils education online. An accomplished researcher with several publications and conference proceedings, Dr. Z currently sits as a peer reviewer for multiple journals. He lives in Atlanta with his wife and four children.